Psychiatry for the Internist

Guest Editor

THEODORE A. STERN, MD

MEDICAL CLINICS
OF NORTH AMERICA

www.medical.theclinics.com

November 2010 • Volume 94 • Number 6

SAUNDERS an imprint of ELSEVIER, Inc.

W.B. SAUNDERS COMPANY
A Division of Elsevier Inc.

1600 John F. Kennedy Boulevard • Suite 1800 • Philadelphia, Pennsylvania 19103-2899

http://www.theclinics.com

MEDICAL CLINICS OF NORTH AMERICA Volume 94, Number 6
November 2010 ISSN 0025-7125, ISBN-13: 978-1-4557-0081-3

Editor: Rachel Glover
Developmental Editor: Donald Mumford

Medical Clinics of North America (ISSN 0025-7125) is published bimonthly by Elsevier Inc., 360 Park Avenue South, New York, NY 10010-1710. Months of issue are January, March, May, July, September, and November. Periodicals postage paid at New York, NY, and additional mailing offices. Subscription prices are USD 218 per year for US individuals, USD 404 per year for US institutions, USD 110 per year for US students, USD 277 per year for Canadian individuals, USD 525 per year for Canadian institutions, USD 173 per year for Canadian students, USD 336 per year for international individuals, USD 525 per year for international institutions and USD 173 per year for international students. To receive student/resident rate, orders must be accompanied by name of affiliated institution, date of term, and the *signature* of program/residency coordinator on institution letterhead. Orders will be billed at individual rate until proof of status is received. Foreign air speed delivery is included in all *Clinics* subscription prices. All prices are subject to change without notice. **POSTMASTER:** Send address changes to *Medical Clinics of North America*, Elsevier Health Sciences Division, Subscription Customer Service, 3251 Riverport Lane, Maryland Heights, MO 63043. **Customer Service: Telephone: 1-800-654-2452** (U.S. and Canada); **1-314-447-8871** (outside U.S. and Canada). **Fax: 1-314-447-8029.** E-mail: **journalscustomerservice-usa@elsevier.com** (for print support); **journalsonlinesupport-usa@elsevier.com** (for online support).

Reprints. For copies of 100 or more of articles in this publication, please contact the Commercial Reprints Department, Elsevier Inc., 360 Park Avenue South, New York, NY 10010-1710. Tel.: 212-633-3812; Fax: 212-462-1935; E-mail: reprints@elsevier.com.

Medical Clinics of North America is also published in Spanish by McGraw-Hill Interamericana Editores S. A., P.O. Box 5-237, 06500 Mexico, D.F., Mexico.

Medical Clinics of North America is covered in *MEDLINE/PubMed (Index Medicus)*, *Current Contents*, *ASCA*, *Excerpta Medica*, *Science Citation Index*, and *ISI/BIOMED*.

Printed in the United States of America.

GOAL STATEMENT
The goal of *Medical Clinics of North America* is to keep practicing physicians up to date with current clinical practice by providing timely articles reviewing the state of the art in patient care.

ACCREDITATION
The *Medical Clinics of North America* is planned and implemented in accordance with the Essential Areas and Policies of the Accreditation Council for Continuing Medical Education (ACCME) through the joint sponsorship of the University of Virginia School of Medicine and Elsevier. The University of Virginia School of Medicine is accredited by the ACCME to provide continuing medical education for physicians.

The University of Virginia School of Medicine designates this educational activity for a maximum of 15 *AMA PRA Category 1 Credits*™ for each issue, 90 credits per year. Physicians should only claim credit commensurate with the extent of their participation in the activity.

The American Medical Association has determined that physicians not licensed in the US who participate in this CME activity are eligible for a maximum of 15 *AMA PRA Category 1 Credits*™ for each issue, 90 credits per year.

Credit can be earned by reading the text material, taking the CME examination online at http://www.theclinics.com/home/cme, and completing the evaluation. After taking the test, you will be required to review any and all incorrect answers. Following completion of the test and evaluation, your credit will be awarded and you may print your certificate.

FACULTY DISCLOSURE/CONFLICT OF INTEREST
The University of Virginia School of Medicine, as an ACCME accredited provider, endorses and strives to comply with the Accreditation Council for Continuing Medical Education (ACCME) Standards of Commercial Support, Commonwealth of Virginia statutes, University of Virginia policies and procedures, and associated federal and private regulations and guidelines on the need for disclosure and monitoring of proprietary and financial interests that may affect the scientific integrity and balance of content delivered in continuing medical education activities under our auspices.

The University of Virginia School of Medicine requires that all CME activities accredited through this institution be developed independently and be scientifically rigorous, balanced and objective in the presentation/discussion of its content, theories and practices.

All authors/editors participating in an accredited CME activity are expected to disclose to the readers relevant financial relationships with commercial entities occurring within the past 12 months (such as grants or research support, employee, consultant, stock holder, member of speakers bureau, etc.). The University of Virginia School of Medicine will employ appropriate mechanisms to resolve potential conflicts of interest to maintain the standards of fair and balanced education to the reader. Questions about specific strategies can be directed to the Office of Continuing Medical Education, University of Virginia School of Medicine, Charlottesville, Virginia.

The faculty and staff of the University of Virginia Office of Continuing Medical Education have no financial affiliations to disclose.

The authors/editors listed below have identified no professional or financial affiliations for themselves or their spouse/partner:
B.J. Beck, MSN, MD; Jason P. Caplan, MD; Catherine C. Crone, MD; Thomas Cummings Jr, MD; Judith G. Edersheim, JD, MD; Steven A. Epstein, MD; Rachel Glover, (Acquisitions Editor); Christopher Gordon, MD; Janna S. Gordon-Elliott, MD; Anne F. Gross, MD; Daniel Hicks, MD; Jeff C. Huffman, MD; Nicholas Kontos, MD; Jose R. Maldonado, MD; Michael J. Marcangelo, MD; Shamim H. Nejad, MD; John Querques, MD; Terry Rabinowitz, MD, DDS; Steven C. Schlozman, MD; Ronald Schouten, MD, JD; Marlynn H. Wei, MD, JD; and Andrew Wolf, MD (Test Author).

The authors/editors listed below identified the following professional or financial affiliations for themselves or their spouse/partner:
Jonathan E. Alpert, MD, PhD receives research support from Abbott Laboratories, Alkermes, Lichtwer Pharma GmbH, Lorex Pharmaceuticals, Aspect Medical Systems, Astra-Zeneca, Bristol-Myers Squibb Company, Cephalon, Cyberonics, Eli Lilly & Company, Forest Pharmaceuticals Inc., GSK, J & J Pharmaceuticals, Novartis, Organon Inc., PamLab, LLC, Pfizer Inc., Pharmavite, Roche, Sanofi/Synthelabo, Solvay Pharaceuticals, Inc., and Wyeth-Ayerst Laboratories; is on the Advisory Committee/Board for Eli Lilly & Company, Pamlab LLC, and Pharmavite LLC.; receives speakers' honoraria from Eli Lilly & Company, Xian-Janssen, Organon, and Reed Medical Education; and receives editorial fees from Belvoir Publishing.
Rebecca Weintraub Brendel, MD, JD is a consultant for Beacon Health Strategies.
Oliver Freudenreich, MD, FAPM is a consultant for Beacon Health Strategies, an industry funded research/investigator for Pfizer, and a speaker for Reed Medical Education.
Philip R. Muskin, MD is on the Speakers' Bureau for AstraZeneca and Bristol-Myers, and is a consultant for Otsuka.
John L. Shuster Jr, MD is an industry funded research/investigator for Abbott Laboratories, Eli Lilly & Co., and Johnson & Johnson.
Theodore A. Stern, MD (Guest Editor) receives royalties for editing for Mosby/Elsevier & McGraw-Hill, receives honorarium for lectures for Reed Elsevier, receives salary for editing Psychosomatics for the Academy of Psychosomatic Medicine, and is a consultant and a stock owner for WiFiMed.

Disclosure of Discussion of Non-FDA Approved Uses for Pharmaceutical Products and/or Medical Devices.
The University of Virginia School of Medicine, as an ACCME provider, requires that all faculty presenters identify and disclose any off-label uses for pharmaceutical and medical device products. The University of Virginia School of Medicine recommends that each physician fully review all the available data on new products or procedures prior to clinical use.

TO ENROLL
To enroll in the Medical Clinics of North America Continuing Medical Education program, call customer service at 1-800-654-2452 or visit us online at http://www.theclinics.com/home/cme. The CME program is available to subscribers for an additional fee of USD 228.

FORTHCOMING ISSUES

RECENT ISSUES

THE CLINICS ARE NOW AVAILABLE ONLINE!

Access your subscription at:
www.theclinics.com

Contributors

GUEST EDITOR

THEODORE A. STERN, MD
Chief, Psychiatric Consultation Service; Director, Office for Clinical Careers,
Massachusetts General Hospital; Professor of Psychiatry of Psychosomatic Medicine,
Harvard Medical School, Boston, Massachusetts

AUTHORS

JONATHAN E. ALPERT, MD, PhD
Associate Chief of Psychiatry for Clinical Services, Associate Professor of Psychiatry,
Harvard Medical School; Associate Director, Depression Clinical and Research
Program; Department of Psychiatry, Massachusetts General Hospital, Boston,
Massachusetts

B.J. BECK, MSN, MD
Assistant Clinical Professor, Department of Psychiatry, Harvard Medical School;
Psychiatrist, Robert B. Andrews Unit, Massachusetts General Hospital, Boston;
Vice President, Medical Affairs, Beacon Health Strategies, LLC, Woburn,
Massachusetts

REBECCA WEINTRAUB BRENDEL, MD, JD
Assistant Professor of Psychiatry, Department of Psychiatry, Massachusetts General
Hospital; Harvard Medical School, Boston, Massachusetts

JASON P. CAPLAN, MD
Chief of Psychiatry, St Joseph's Hospital and Medical Center, Phoenix,
Arizona; Vice-Chair of Psychiatry, Creighton University School of Medicine,
Omaha, Nebraska

CATHERINE C. CRONE, MD
Associate Professor, Department of Psychiatry, George Washington University,
Washington, DC; Clinical Professor, Department of Psychiatry, Northern Virginia Branch,
Virginia Commonwealth University, Richmond; Department of Psychiatry, Inova Fairfax
Hospital, Falls Church, Virginia

THOMAS CUMMINGS Jr, MD
Assistant Professor and Associate Director, Inpatient Psychiatry, Department
of Psychiatry, Georgetown University Hospital and School of Medicine,
Washington, DC

JUDITH G. EDERSHEIM, JD, MD
Instructor, Harvard Medical School; Senior Consultant, Law and Psychiatry Service,
Department of Psychiatry, Massachusetts General Hospital, Boston, Massachusetts

STEVEN A. EPSTEIN, MD
Professor and Chair, Department of Psychiatry, Georgetown University Hospital and School of Medicine, Washington, DC

OLIVER FREUDENREICH, MD, FAPM
Assistant Professor of Psychiatry, Harvard Medical School; Director, Infectious Disease Psychiatric Consultation Service; Division of Psychiatry and Medicine, Department of Medicine, Massachusetts General Hospital, Boston, Massachusetts

CHRISTOPHER GORDON, MD
Assistant Clinical Professor, Department of Psychiatry, Harvard Medical School, Boston; Vice President, Clinical Services and Medical Director, Advocates, Inc, Framingham; Assistant Psychiatrist, Department of Psychiatry, Massachusetts General Hospital, Boston, Massachusetts

JANNA S. GORDON-ELLIOTT, MD
Post-Graduate Clinical Fellow in Psychosomatic Medicine, New York State Psychiatric Institute, Department of Psychiatry, New York-Presbyterian Hospital, Columbia University Medical Center, New York, New York

ANNE F. GROSS, MD
Clinical Fellow in Psychiatry, Harvard Medical School; Resident in Psychiatry Massachusetts General Hospital/McLean Psychiatry Residency Program, Massachusetts General Hospital, Boston, Massachusetts

DANIEL HICKS, MD
Associate Professor and Director, Psychosomatic Medicine Service, Department of Psychiatry, Georgetown University Hospital and School of Medicine, Washington, DC

JEFF C. HUFFMAN, MD
Medical Director, Inpatient Psychiatry, Massachusetts General Hospital; Assistant Professor of Psychiatry, Harvard Medical School, Boston, Massachusetts

NICHOLAS KONTOS, MD
Director, Transplantation Psychiatry, Department of Psychiatry, Massachusetts General Hospital; Instructor in Psychiatry, Harvard Medical School, Boston, Massachusetts

JOSE R. MALDONADO, MD, FAPM, FACFE
Associate Professor of Psychiatry, Medicine and Surgery; Medical Director, Psychosomatic Medicine Service; Chief, Medical Psychotherapy Clinic, Stanford University School of Medicine, Stanford, California

MICHAEL J. MARCANGELO, MD
Assistant Professor and Director of Medical Student Education, Department of Psychiatry and Behavioral Neuroscience, University of Chicago Hospitals, Chicago, Illinois

PHILIP R. MUSKIN, MD
Professor of Clinical Psychiatry, Department of Psychiatry, Columbia University College of Physicians and Surgeons; Chief of Service, Division of Consultation-Liaison Psychiatry, New York-Presbyterian Hospital, Columbia University Medical Center; Faculty Psychoanalyst, Columbia University Psychoanalytic Center for Research and Training, New York, New York

SHAMIM H. NEJAD, MD
Instructor in Psychiatry, Harvard Medical School; Director, Adult Burns and Trauma Surgery Consultation; Division of Psychiatry and Medicine, Department of Psychiatry, Massachusetts General Hospital, Boston, Massachusetts

JOHN QUERQUES, MD
Associate Director, Psychosomatic Medicine-Consultation Psychiatry Fellowship Program, Department of Psychiatry, Massachusetts General Hospital; Assistant Professor of Psychiatry, Harvard Medical School, Boston, Massachusetts

TERRY RABINOWITZ, MD, DDS
Professor of Psychiatry and Family Medicine; Medical Director, Division of Consultation Psychiatry and Psychosomatic Medicine; Medical Director, Telemedicine; University of Vermont College of Medicine; Fletcher Allen Health Care, Burlington, Vermont

STEVEN C. SCHLOZMAN, MD
Co-Director, Medical Student Education in Psychiatry, Assistant Professor of Psychiatry, Harvard Medical School; Associate Director, Child and Adolescent Psychiatry Residency, Staff Child Psychiatrist, Massachusetts General Hospital/McLean Program in Child Psychiatry; Harvard Graduate School of Education, Massachusetts General Hospital, Boston, Massachusetts

RONALD SCHOUTEN, MD, JD
Department of Psychiatry, Massachusetts General Hospital; Harvard Medical School, Boston, Massachusetts

JOHN L. SHUSTER Jr, MD
Professor of Psychiatry and Medicine and Director, Psychiatry and Medicine Program, Department of Psychiatry, Vanderbilt University School of Medicine, Nashville, Tennessee

MARLYNN H. WEI, MD, JD
Consult-Liaison Psychiatry and Administrative Chief Resident, Clinical Fellow in Psychiatry, Massachusetts General Hospital; Harvard Medical School, Boston, Massachusetts

Contents

Although changes in the US health care system promote a population-based approach, increases in population diversity emphasize the need for culturally competent, patient-centered, participatory care. Despite this perceived conflict, the global view has improved the recognition of mental health issues as a driver of overall health as well as health care spending. This recognition, along with the many forces that keep mental health care in the primary care sector, actually encourages the development of collaborative models that capitalize on the primary care provider's opportunity to leverage their rapport with the patient to improve access to, and comfort with, specialty mental health services. Engaging patients in their own path to recovery or well-being improves engagement in, and adherence to, the treatment plan and ultimately improves outcomes.

Suicide is one of the leading causes of death in the United States and is defined as intentional self-harm with the intent of causing death. Various mental disorders may be a cause for increased violence. This article outlines the elements of the risk assessment (for harm to self and/or others) in patients in crisis and addresses which contributing factors may be modifiable. This article also proposes a practical framework for the management of risk regarding suicide and violence.

Patients with cognitive impairment can be divided into 2 broad groups: those with chronic cognitive decline (most likely diagnosable with a dementia) and those with acute cognitive changes (most likely experiencing a delirium). However, diagnosis in clinical practice is far more complicated than it is in textbooks. Perhaps the greatest hurdle in evaluating the cognitively impaired patient is the clarification of a cohesive history. Unfortunately, the cognitively impaired patient is most often unable to provide such a history, and in the absence of a reliable family member, friend, or caregiver to fill in the gaps, diagnostic clarity can be difficult to achieve. This article outlines the broad diagnostic spectra of delirium and dementia, reviews current understanding of their pathogenesis, and discusses useful diagnostic and therapeutic techniques.

Americans aged 12 years or older (8% of the US population) had used an illicit drug during the preceding month. Some licit substances also create havoc. The survey found that slightly more than half (56%) of Americans reported being current drinkers of alcohol. A total of 6.2 million (2.5%) Americans used prescription-type psychotherapeutic drugs for nonmedical purposes and 70.9 million Americans (or 28.4%) used tobacco during the survey period. Substance abuse problems were diagnosed in up to 36% of medically hospitalized patients for whom a psychiatric consultation was requested. Given how prevalent the use of substances is among the medically ill and their potential effect on comorbid medical conditions, it is important for physicians to be mindful of their prevalence and presentation. This article covers the presenting symptoms of intoxication and withdrawal states, addresses the acute management of the most commonly encountered substances, and summarizes all others in a table.

Doctors diagnose and treat disease; illness is the experience of, and response to, a disease by patients and the people in their lives. Discrepancies between disease and illness (eg, adjustment to the sick role, treatment-related difficulties, denial of medical illness, and psychiatric comorbidity) are prevalent, as are somatoform disorders and other conditions in which patients are invested in being understood as medically ill. This article reviews suggestions for physicians' responses to these patients and their dilemmas.

Primary care physicians commonly deal with patients who present with a somatic complaint for which no clear organic etiology can be found. This article discusses how a psychiatrist thinks about somatic symptoms (eg, pain, insomnia, weight loss and loss of appetite, fatigue and forgetfulness, sexual dysfunction) in a patient who might have depression. The management of a patient in whom no satisfactory medical or psychiatric diagnosis can be made is also reviewed briefly.

Medical practice occurs within a legal and regulatory context. This article covers several of the legal issues that frequently arise in the general medical setting. While this article provides an overview of approaches to informed consent, boundary issues, and malpractice claims, it is critical for clinicians to be familiar with the specific requirements and standards in the jurisdictions in which they practice. As a general rule, it is most important that physicians recognize that the best way to avoid legal problems is to be aware of legal requirements in the jurisdictions in which they practice, but to think clinically and not legally in the provision of consistent and sound clinical care to their patients.

Organ transplantation offers an opportunity for extended survival and enhanced quality of life to patients with end-stage organ disease. Significant challenges are associated with both pre- and post-transplantation care, however, that require awareness of psychiatric issues in this patient population. Ventricular assist devices have added another dimension to patient care and to quality-of-life considerations. Unfortunately, effective incorporation of palliative care and end-of-life discussions is frequently overlooked during caretaking of these patients.

Preface

Psychiatry for the Internist

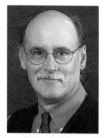

Theodore A. Stern, MD
Guest Editor

Some clinicians may wonder why a special issue devoted to psychiatry for the internist is needed, as so much of an internist's daily practice involves psychiatric issues. However, familiarity with problems does not always equate with expertise or even comfort and/or competence. Therefore, this volume aims to review reasonable approaches to common psychiatric conditions and situations and to guide thoughtful strategies and informed interventions. The core jobs of an internist, to diagnose and to treat, are often complex and conducted under the pressure of time. This leads some practitioners to target the "low-hanging fruit" of patient problems and to prioritize concerns (so as not to get bogged down in a quagmire of dilemmas and complaints). Unfortunately, psychiatric conditions are among those most often linked with disability days and dysphoria; addressing psychiatric diagnoses and their manifestations will increase patient satisfaction and decrease dysfunction and overall health care costs.

This volume starts off with an informed discussion of an approach to collaborative care and cultural competence and then proceeds to the assessment of patients in crisis (providing pointers for the determination of the risks of suicide and/or violence). Then, approaches to patients with cognitive dysfunction (eg, with delirium or dementia), dysregulated mood (eg, major depressive disorder, bipolar disorder), and anxiety are offered. Treatment strategies, involving pharmacological (eg, use of antidepressants, antipsychotics, anxiolytics, mood stabilizers, natural remedies) and non-pharmacological approaches (eg, talking therapies), are reviewed. Chronic diseases (eg, substance use and abuse, somatoform disorders, cancer, diabetes, sleep disturbances, gastrointestinal distress, premenstrual dysphoria) and their management are then discussed. Forensic issues (eg, approaches to informed consent, capacity decisions, civil commitment, malpractice, boundary crossings) are reviewed to inform clinicians about necessary knowledge and responsibilities. The volume ends with a discussion of end-of-life treatment decisions and organ failure/transplantation. For further information on these and other topics, relevant to your practice, useful references are available.[1–4]

Med Clin N Am 94 (2010) xiii–xiv
doi:10.1016/j.mcna.2010.08.036
0025-7125/10/$ – see front matter © 2010 Elsevier Inc. All rights reserved.

medical.theclinics.com

It is our sincere hope that the presentation of these common conditions and problematic issues is readable, informative, and helpful to you and to your patients.

Theodore A. Stern, MD
Massachusetts General Hospital
Harvard Medical School
55 Fruit Street
Warren Building, Room 605
Boston, MA 02114, USA

E-mail address:
TStern@partners.org

REFERENCES

1. Stern TA, Herman JB, Slavin PL, editors. The Massachusetts General Hospital Guide to primary care psychiatry. 2nd edition. New York: McGraw-Hill; 2004 (also produced in Spanish language edition 2005; Madrid).
2. Stern TA, editor. The ten-minute guide to psychiatric diagnosis and treatment. New York: Professional Publishing Group; 2005.
3. Stern TA, Rosenbaum JF, Fava M, et al, editors. Massachusetts General Hospital comprehensive clinical psychiatry. Philadelphia (PA): Mosby/Elsevier; 2008.
4. Stern TA, Fricchione G, Cassem NH, et al, editors. Massachusetts General Hospital handbook of general hospital psychiatry. 6th edition. Philadelphia (PA): Saunders/Elsevier; 2010.

An Approach to Collaborative Care and Consultation: Interviewing, Cultural Competence, and Enhancing Rapport and Adherence

B.J. Beck, MSN, MD[a,b,c],*, Christopher Gordon, MD[a,d,e]

KEYWORDS

- Collaborative care • Cultural competence • Rapport
- Adherence • Primary care • Consultation psychiatry

Parallel trends in American mental[1] and physical[2] healthcare over the last century have created a complex, discontinuous, and fragmented system of outpatient services to care for increasingly diverse and seriously ill patient populations. Starting with deinstitutionalization in the 1950s[3] and continuing with the managed care movement in the early 1990s, the locus of psychiatric care, even for the most severely ill, is community based, rather than hospital based (although community resources have not kept pace with the growing need). This mode of care correlates with the trend toward shorter hospital stays for medical and surgical conditions, shifting the locus of many

The authors have nothing to disclose.

[a] Department of Psychiatry, Harvard Medical School, 25 Shattuck Street, Boston, MA 02115, USA

[b] Robert B. Andrews Unit, Massachusetts General Hospital, 15 Parkman, Boston, MA 02114, USA

[c] Medical Affairs, Beacon Health Strategies, LLC, 500 Unicorn Park Drive #401, Woburn, MA 01801, USA

[d] Advocates, Inc, One Clarks Hill, Suite 305, Framingham, MA 01702, USA

[e] Department of Psychiatry, Massachusetts General Hospital, 15 Parkman, Boston, MA 02114, USA

* Corresponding author. Department of Psychiatry, Massachusetts General Hospital, ACC 812, 15 Parkman Street, Boston, MA 02114.

E-mail address: bbeck@partners.org

Med Clin N Am 94 (2010) 1075–1088

doi:10.1016/j.mcna.2010.08.001

0025-7125/10/$ – see front matter © 2010 Elsevier Inc. All rights reserved.

consultation psychiatrists from the inpatient to the outpatient arena. The general medical setting has long been the de facto mental health system for those with less severe or disabling symptoms.[4] Not until 2002 did slightly more (55.1%) US community dwellers seek care in the mental health (rather than the physical health) system for depression, the most common primary care psychiatric disorder.[5] Nonetheless, patients in primary care continue to be highly symptomatic and distressed.

Many patients continue to prefer that their mental health needs be addressed in the primary care setting for a variety of reasons (eg, stigma, shame, financial and other barriers to specialty care access). For an equally enduring set of reasons (eg, time constraints, productivity demands, limited training, minimal referral resources), primary care providers (PCPs) have been reluctant to recognize what they feel ill-equipped to treat and unable to refer easily.[6–8] Some PCPs also share their patients' sense of stigma; they often worry that patients will feel insulted by having a psychiatric diagnosis. Adding to this disconnect is the reality that patients who present to primary care settings are different from those who seek care in specialty clinics. Primary care patients tend to present earlier, with somatic rather than mental/emotional complaints, and often have a great deal of distress without meeting criteria for a diagnosable disorder (ie, they have subsyndromal symptoms).[9]

More recent studies have shown that PCPs recognize the more severely depressed[10] or anxious[11] patients in their practices and that less severely affected primary care patients often do quite well on relatively inadequate (ie, short and low dose) trials of selective serotonin reuptake inhibitors.[8,10] As the medications used to treat the common primary care psychiatric disorders have become safer, more tolerable, and easier to use, more PCPs have been willing to prescribe them for their symptomatic patients.[12] Possibly because of these generally good outcomes, prescriptive practice of PCPs has not routinely been accompanied by appropriate monitoring for side effects, therapeutic outcome, or the need for medication titration.[13]

At present, the more serious mental health conditions are recognized in primary care, and there are effective evidence-based treatments and treatment guidelines; however, some patients are being prescribed appropriate medications but are not improving.[5] Even when unarguably necessary, the prescription itself is not sufficient. A patient's genetic, cultural, and linguistic factors converge to determine the efficacy of a given prescription (eg, whether it is filled, how and when it is taken).[14] The effect of cultural beliefs and expectations on treatment adherence may be more pertinent to treatment outcome than that of the actual modality, medication, or dose prescribed.[15]

These individual and cultural influences on adherence are at odds with the necessary trend toward population-based (as opposed to patient-based) care to address the rapid escalation in health care costs. The patients most affected and most in need (eg, ethnic and racial minorities, non-English speaking patients, women, the elderly,[12,16] and those struggling with addictions) are least able to trust, navigate, or advocate for themselves in this fragmented and discontinuous system. Yet, a more global view of population-based care has shed light on the tremendous overall cost of psychiatric morbidity (including increased physical health care costs,[17,18] increased work absenteeism, presenteeism,[19] higher unemployment rates, disability,[20] and even mortality). Soon to be a reality, true parity is long overdue.

However, regardless of the system or trends, the primary care challenge remains to recognize and treat the patient's distress (in a culturally acceptable manner that incorporates the patient's beliefs, expectations, social environment, and personal engagement and does not overly disrupt the PCP's workflow). The nature of primary care is such that PCPs have the opportunity to know a great deal about their patients, including their cultural view and beliefs, and patients have the opportunity to develop a sense of trust, or rapport, with their PCPs (around issues possibly less threatening than their mental health). This cultural information, and seasoned relationship, gathered over time through multiple observations and conversations is key to personalizing a guideline-informed approach to the treatment of the more common primary care mental health conditions. This relationship paves the way for a collaborative approach that builds a therapeutic alliance and engages the patient in treatment decisions.

A collaborative relationship with a psychiatric specialist, for focused training and consultation, can also help the PCP to leverage their extensive patient experience to best meet the patients' mental health needs in the setting of the patients' greatest comfort, the PCP's office. When the patient's condition is beyond the appropriate expertise of the PCP, this relationship and the PCP's rapport with the patient also enhance the referral process. This increases the odds of a successful new treatment alliance, with communication and coordination between all members of the patient's treatment team.

CULTURAL COMPETENCE AND COLLABORATIVE CONSULTATION

Most patients, across cultures, ethnicities, and languages, prefer patient-centered care (ie, care that engages the patient as an expert partner in a collaborative project to determine an optimal path toward wellness, recovery, and disease management).[21] Patient-centered care consistently yields better health outcomes, higher patient satisfaction, lower malpractice claims, greater adherence to treatment protocols, and greater longevity of patient-doctor relationships.[22–27] Patient-centered care (also called participatory or relationship-centered care[28]) embodies the primary care values of caring for the whole person in a lifelong process to promote health and well-being.[27] Ideal patient-centered care is culturally competent; when immediate cultural familiarity and knowledge are not practical, the practitioner must practice cultural humility.[29]

Patient-centered participatory care is particularly important and effective in delivering mental health care in the primary care setting. Patients who enjoy a collaborative secure relationship with their primary care doctors are more likely to surface mental health issues and to be receptive to proffered treatments.[30]

CLINICAL INTERVIEWING, WITH SPECIAL REFERENCE TO POSSIBLE MENTAL HEALTH CONDITIONS

An effective interview creates an atmosphere of mutuality, respect, interest, and care in which patients feel welcome, safe, and understood from their own perspective.[31] In this relationship, patient and doctor come together as mutual experts, the physician as an expert in health, wellness, disease, recovery, and disease management and the patient as an expert in their own body, life, values, preferences, hopes, and concerns. To the extent that the patient is an expert in their own life, the relationship of the doctor to the patient is, in this aspect, one of a student to a teacher.[29] Out of this partnership between experts, a mutually designed path and mutually determined choices in treatment create the best chance for treatment adherence, optimal clinical outcomes, and longevity and vitality of the relationship itself. Among its many benefits, this partnership negates the power differential between physician and patient. Such a differential, as discussed later, is particularly salient for patients of minority cultures and contributes insidiously to patients feeling unengaged in their treatment planning and ultimately to nonadherence and poor outcomes.[32]

The physicians' appreciation for the patients' culture (eg, ethnicity, language, gender, sexual orientation, other culturally significant qualities) is central to the patients' feeling of being understood on their own terms (ie, feeling understood as one understands one's self).[33] In addition to openness and respect for the patient's culture, demonstrable as well as technical knowledge and expertise, other qualities sought by most patients in this partnering relationship are confidence, humane warmth, a personal approach, forthrightness, thoroughness, and a commitment to delivering on promises.[21]

The *sine qua non* of effective clinical interviewing, as for the relationship as a whole, is rapport: that feeling of chemistry between people, that reflects the sense of being understood, accepted, comfortable, and at ease.[28,31] The first and most critical goal of the interview is to foster and nurture rapport. With rapport, much is possible, such as crafting a working plan that the patients endorse as their own. With rapport, conflicts and disagreements about the nature of the problem, the path of treatment, or other aspects of the doctor-patient relationship can be dealt with smoothly and explicitly. Without rapport, the outcome of the work and the relationship itself are in peril; conflicts go unspoken and often unacknowledged and may surface as nonadherence or noncompliance and end in bad outcomes.

BUILDING A HISTORY

One of the most important ingredients in effective interviewing, and one in terribly short supply, is time.[31] Sufficient time to comfortably welcome the patient, and not rush through the interview, is an uncommon luxury in many clinical settings. Nonetheless, physicians are particularly prone to empathy-destroying and relationship-harming behaviors (eg, cutting the patient off, frequent interruptions, asking too many closed-ended or symptom-linked questions, and generally doing too much of the talking).[34] Research suggests that investing time up front in effective partnership ultimately saves time.[23] The overarching goals of the clinical interview are not only to identify the patients' key problems, but to get to know them as a whole, contextualized in their strengths, relationships, history, and attitudes.[35]

At the beginning of the interview, the immediate goal is to create an atmosphere conducive to rapport. "Getting the nod"[36] is a good barometer for successful rapport building at this phase. That is, as the physician summarizes their understanding of the patient's opening narrative, the patient nods in assent.[28] One very good way to accomplish this is for the physician to offer to tell the patient what the physician already know about them. This maneuver may seem counterintuitive because it does involve the physician doing the initial talking. However, the advantages of this maneuver are that (1) the doctor "shows their cards" first and open the way for the patient to correct misinformation and (2) it offers the physician a way to briefly summarize the information in a friendly welcoming way. Moreover, by asking the patient's permission to relate this information, the power in the relationship immediately shifts from doctor to patient.[28,37]

Next, it is important that the physician listens to whatever follows this opening, with open ears, heart, and mind. Physicians need to stifle the impulse to interrupt and need to encourage the person with nonverbal supports, such as leaning forward, nodding, and providing gentle introjections (such as "I see" or "how difficult") at appropriate times.[25] After listening in this active way, at a reasonable pause point, it is advisable for the physicians to reflect what they have heard. A good technique for this is to ask permission, "May I see if I understand clearly what you have been saying so far?" This permission seeking is another power-shifting statement and pulls again for a nod.[37] Summarizing in a nod-worthy manner is a clinical art.[28] What is reflected back must feel right, familiar, and sensible to the patient, which is more likely to occur by using the patient's exact key words. Rapport is further fostered by clinical transparency or guided interviewing in which the physician explains what they are asking about while moving through the interview.[28,36] Simple explanations cue the patient as to the sort of information being sought and demystify the process of the interview.

In this manner, the history of the present illness is fleshed out, with the patient and doctor having a common perception of the current issues or problem. The remainder of the history taking, or, more collaboratively, history building,[38] involves placing the current problem in the context of the person's psychiatric history, medical history, social and developmental context, as well as strengths and capacities. For some patients, a formal mental status examination of cognition, memory, or other intellectual functions may be necessary; but most of the mental status examination in a primary care setting can be inferred.

The social and developmental histories are particularly rich sources of information for getting to know the patient as a whole person. Questions may range from "Whom do you live with now?" to "What is life like at home?" or "Who are the most important people in your life now?" A particularly deep and effective probe is to ask, "What was it like for you growing up?"

It is also very important to not lose sight of the person's strengths, talents, and accomplishments as the physician learns about the suffering and difficulty in the person's life. Asking about hobbies, interests, passions, things that the person either does now or once did for fun, and hopes and dreams for the future can be wonderful windows into this part of the person's selfhood.[28] Similarly, it is important to appreciate the person's religious or spiritual orientation or practice.

When the interviewer feels the history building is close to completion, it is wise to ask whether there is anything the patient would like to add or emphasize.[37] However, if it is not clear at this point, it is useful to ask the patient how they were hoping the doctor might be able to help them, and whether they have any worries or concerns about what the doctor might offer.

DISCUSSING THE PROBLEM

At this point, the physician should be able to summarize their shared understanding of the patient's key issues. In order to discuss the problem and to move toward a path of treatment, the physician must bear in mind the difference between diagnosis and formulation. Psychiatric diagnoses, even to psychiatrists themselves, can seem flat, nondescriptive of the situation, oversimplified, and less than useful in constructing comprehensive and effective paths toward recovery. To tell patients that they have major depression is to use a term that is ambiguous and may be very frightening, upsetting, and off-putting.[39] A formulation contextualizes the problem and paints a picture of the real human being contending with life's challenges, including what may or may not be a discrete diagnosis.[28]

One excellent model for contextualizing challenges in a manner that is accessible to patients is to use the bio-psycho-social-spiritual model. The order may be slightly changed in clinical practice. An effective way of using this model is to offer to share with the patient how physicians think about people, as follows[28]:

"I wonder if it would be all right with you, before we get into talking about what we can do to help you, if I would share with you how I think about people in my work as a psychiatrist? In general, I think about everyone who is having troubles from four points of view. Then I try to put these four points of view together to see if any of them might be helpful. The first point of view is a social one—basically, is there something going on in the here-and-now world of living that is really hurting this person? It could be a husband who is lying, or it could be a sick child, or not having enough money. The key is that it is happening here and now. The

second model I think about is a biologic perspective—could some part of this problem be due to a chemical imbalance of some sort—like a thyroid problem, or sometimes certain kinds of depression or anxiety are caused by chemical imbalances. The third model is psychological, and by that I mean that every person I ever knew has baggage from the past, and sometimes it is the baggage from the past that is making life now very hard. And the last way I think about people, which is not applicable to everyone but is really important for some people, is spiritual; is something going on in this person's spiritual life, like they had faith and lost it, or something else is happening that is making life seem empty of meaning. Do these models make sense to you?"

Most people resonate with and can relate to the 4 models. These models are particularly useful because they are nonpathologizing and are rather universal about human difficulties. By asking the person which, if any, of these models seems to make the most sense in understanding their particular difficulty, a fruitful and mutual discussion about a path forward can be promoted.

BUILDING A PATH FORWARD

These 4 models lend themselves very well to teasing out biologic aspects of the problem (which may be treatable with psychiatric medications) without overemphasizing the role of medications in addressing other challenges (like marital infidelity). The 4 models are also very flexible with regard to appreciating cultural and ethnic aspects of the patient's experience. These models also blend easily with natural supports and strengths.[40]

CULTURAL COMPETENCE AND COLLABORATIVE CARE

The model of clinical interviewing outlined earlier can engage the whole person in a collaborative process of understanding the patient's situation, concerns, and preferences and for co-creating a path toward health. This approach actively incorporates awareness of the patient's cultural heritage and milieu as it bears on their current experience.[41]

Following Betancourt and colleagues,[42] culture is defined as "an integrated pattern of learned beliefs and behaviors that can be shared among groups…(which) includes thoughts, styles of communicating, ways of interacting, views on roles and relationships, values, practices and customs…shaped by many influences including race, ethnicity, nationality, language, and gender, as well as socioeconomic status, physical and mental ability, sexual orientation and occupation," among other traits. Cultural competence denotes a capability by a health system, or a practitioner or team within it, to render care that meets the needs of patients with diverse values, beliefs, and behaviors, tailoring care to meet patients' diverse social, cultural, and linguistic needs.[42]

Such cultural competence is of growing importance because the diversity of the population in the United States continues to increase.[29] Individuals from nonmajority cultural groups often report less satisfaction with health care treatment, less experience of participatory decision making with their practitioners, and less experience of overall trust with their practitioners.[41] These disparities increase with discordance, racial, ethnic, or linguistic, between doctor-patient pairs and seem to be further increased in populations who have experienced discrimination, for example, African Americans.[41]

Efforts to increase cultural competence can include (1) staff training on cultural differences and their associated health disparities, as well as introductions to important belief systems, values, practices, and other norms in communities in which the team operates, (2) active recruitment and mentoring of minority staff in all positions, (3) active and substantial support to ensure professional translation and interpretation services, (4) provision of teaching and other materials in language and formats congenial to the population, (5) active recruitment of minority community members for representation on boards of directors and other roles in program evaluation and design, and (6) active use of patient satisfaction surveys, with feedback to treatment teams with time for analysis and reflection.[42]

Even with these activities, true cultural competence is always more a goal than a reality. Every individual, by virtue of the many roles that they play in the world, may be a member of numerous cultures, defined by gender, race, language, ethnicity, sexual orientation, class, disability, and so on. So it has been suggested that what is desirable is cultural humility, and flexibility, and that the process of achieving cultural competence is a lifelong commitment to learning, with each other, with patients, with the community, and with ourselves.[29,42]

Physicians can find ways to more deeply understand and collaborate with patients by being aware of cultural differences. By understanding that people from minority cultures often bring with them previous less-than-optimal experiences with health care professionals, physicians can redouble their efforts to practice collaborative medicine and shared decision making, aware of and sensitive to the power differentials between doctor and patient that can be aggravated by cultural discordance within the doctor-patient dyad.[32]

ADHERENCE AND CULTURAL COMPETENCE

Nonadherence to treatment recommendations is ubiquitous in health care, profoundly expensive, and multifactorial.[43] An estimated 85% of patients are at times nonadherent to treatment recommendations,[44] with the annual cost of nonadherence close to 100 billion dollars.[44] Even with respect to such lifesaving and relatively side effect–benign treatments (eg, statins, antihypertensives), adherence rates are no better than about 50%. With respect to lifestyle recommendations (eg, diet, exercise), adherence is much worse, with successful outcomes of perhaps 10%.[43] Nonadherence is hard to measure in daily practice but must always be considered with less-than-optimal outcomes. Nonadherence is also significantly underreported; acknowledging even missing any medication as prescribed probably translates in reality to less than 60% adherence.[43]

Many factors contribute to nonadherence. These factors range from the patient's rational response to inadequate, unclear, or unconvincing information from their practitioner, to other factors in the doctor-patient relationship (such as disagreement over the nature of the problem to be solved or the treatment designed to deal with it). Other factors that significantly contribute to nonadherence are cost, medication side effects, complex medication regimens, significant improvement in symptoms without treatment, and misunderstanding about the regimen to be followed.[44,45] Nonadherence is a particularly vexing problem with regard to psychiatric treatment recommendations in primary care. Although most psychiatric medications are prescribed in the primary care setting, their adherence rates are about 40% for reasons previously detailed, and the additional difficulty of patient-doctor disagreement about the mental versus the physical nature of the condition and the stigma associated with mental health conditions and their treatment.[30]

The best approach to treatment nonadherence is to develop a participatory decision-making structure in the clinical practice.[45] Participatory collaborative decision making minimizes the chance that doctor and patient have an unstated disagreement about the nature of the problem and the best path for its treatment.[46] Moreover, nonparticipatory decision making pulls for upstream decisional uncertainty and patient reservations, which if left undiscussed and unacknowledged, could later blossom into nonadherence, often only to be discovered after more serious problems have evolved.[47,48]

COLLABORATION

To effectively address and treat mental health issues in primary care, collaboration pertains to the patient-PCP relationship and also rightfully extends to the PCP-consultant psychiatrist relationship. The purpose of PCP-specialist collaboration is 4-fold: to improve access, treatment, outcomes, and communication. Much has already been stated about the patient's preference for the primary care setting, but this collaborative relationship with a psychiatric expert has benefit for the PCP as well. The ready access to the specialist removes the onus of recognizing something that the PCP feels ill-prepared to treat or refer. Such access also emboldens the PCP to initiate treatment for those mental health conditions that truly are the rightful domain of primary care (eg, depression and anxiety disorders), knowing that advice, consultation, or referral is available as necessary. This opportunity for real-time consultation increases the likelihood of adequate and effective treatment.

Not all patients or their mental health issues are appropriate for primary care management. However, the collaborative PCP is in the ideal position to leverage their rapport with their patient to facilitate the patient's willing acceptance of a referral to, or consultation with, the psychiatrist, improving access to specialty care when needed. There are also studies of collaborative models in which the PCP and psychiatrist alternate visits[49,50] in a more expensive, but more effective and cost-effective,[51] treatment for more seriously depressed patients, who would not otherwise be appropriate for primary care mental health management.[52–54] But perhaps most significant for the PCP, as well as for the quality and coordination of the patient's total care, is the eradication of the black box approach that has all too long prevailed over referral mental health treatment. A true collaboration means that the PCPs and specialists are within the circle of care, with reciprocal flow of pertinent clinical information and the respectful recognition of the PCP as the broker of all specialty care and services in the agreed upon treatment plan of their patient.

PREPARATION FOR SUCCESSFUL COLLABORATION

It is worth the time necessary to define the roles and expectations relevant to the chosen model to avoid misunderstandings that might undermine the effective collaboration or rapport between patient and PCP or between patient and psychiatrist. For instance, all parties should understand that the PCP is the hub of the circle of care, and brokers all services on the patient's behalf. The psychiatrist may be a consultant to the PCP or an intermittent treater or cotreater. If the psychiatrist is to see the patient, the patient should have a clear understanding of what to expect, in terms of the relationship with the psychiatrist (eg, will this be a 1-time consultation or will there be ongoing treatment?) as well as the content of the visit (ie, what to expect in a psychiatric appointment is not intuitive and much scary folklore persists). The psychiatrist should also state and clarify, as necessary, the nature and parameters of the visit(s).

Confidentiality is also worth an up-front discussion. If the psychiatrist is a consultant to the PCP and within the circle of care, the patient should be aware of the intent to share communication between the psychiatrist and PCP. Just as there are limits to confidentiality in private practice (eg, suicidal ideation), there may be respectful limits to shared communication (eg, a woman who discloses childhood incest may not want this in her medical record; the psychiatrist might accommodate that request in a way that shares the pertinent information, "patient experienced a childhood trauma"). If the PCP and psychiatrist are not truly within the systematic circle of care, the patient should sign releases to allow for communication, an act that further objectifies this intention.

Collaboration requires education. The specialist has a commitment to provide pragmatic information to the PCP who is expected to participate in the mental health treatment of their patient. This information may be provided in an informal manner (a curbside consultation), as written explanations in consultation notes, or via more formal (continuing medical education [CME]–type) seminars or presentations. The PCP must educate the specialist on issues of their practice and workflow. Any clinician who meets with the patient has a responsibility to educate the patient about the clinician's role and to demystify their process. And, as previously mentioned, doctors need to listen for the patient to educate them about the patient's life, culture, beliefs, fears and aspirations.

COLLABORATIVE MODELS TO ADDRESS THE CHALLENGES OF PRIMARY CARE

A variety of innovative models developed over the past several decades differ in some key features that make these models more or less appropriate for particular medical settings.[55] These differentiating features include where and whether the patient is seen by the psychiatrist; whether there is a 1-time consultation, a few visits, or ongoing care; whether there are shared records; how providers communicate with each other; and whether there is an ongoing relationship between the PCP and psychiatrist. Beyond these features, the successful model must also accommodate the tremendous constraints and demands of the twenty-first century primary care practice, respecting and addressing issues such as space, time, payment, ancillary support, and available community services. The 3 models chosen for brief description (discussed later) are truly collaborative and respectful of these primary care pressures.

Each model has several underlying, implicit or explicit, assumptions. These collaborative models share several assumptions. They all assume that mental health issues for some patients can be adequately and appropriately cared for in the primary care setting, the collaborative PCP-specialist relationship enhances that care, and communication is essential because the PCP is responsible for the patient's total care. These models also assume the need for education and a multidisciplinary team approach. Implicit assumptions are that PCPs can most reasonably be expected to participate in the medical (ie, medication) management of mental health disorders and that other resources are necessary for other (more time-consuming) treatment modalities.

COLLABORATIVE MANAGEMENT

In collaborative care, patients initially alternate visits between the PCP and psychiatrist, within the primary care clinic.[49–54,56] PCPs receive training at the outset and continue to participate in ongoing teaching conferences. Rigorously studied for persistent and late-life depression and panic disorder, this intensive model is cost-effective for more seriously affected patients who might otherwise need ongoing specialty care. Hence, patients are generally referred by their PCPs after failing a more standard trial of primary care treatment (ie, one or more unsuccessful medication trials). There is an educational component for patients as well as a specific type of short-term therapy with a trained office nurse, supervised by the psychiatrist. An obvious benefit of the model is the patient's ability to receive quality care in the primary care setting, with ongoing contact and rapport with their trusted PCP who is able to relay their extensive understanding of the patient as a whole person to the collaborating psychiatrist.

THE 3-COMPONENT MODEL

The MacArthur Initiative on Depression in Primary Care promoted the development of the Three Component Model (TCM),[57] which adds infrastructure to the consultative collaboration, relies heavily on the team approach, has built-in outcomes and adherence measures, and maximizes the number of appropriately cared for patients in the primary care setting. In this model, depression is viewed and treated like other chronic illnesses that require ongoing management. The 3 components of the TCM are the PCP, psychiatrist, and care manager. Written and electronic training and educational modules exist for all participants, the PCP, psychiatrist, care manager, and patient. The care protocol roughly follows common evidence-based depression treatment guidelines. Although the psychiatrist may occasionally evaluate a patient, most of the psychiatric consultation is telephonic with the care manager, who is generally a nurse in the practice. The (primarily phone based) care manager is the vector for communication and coordination, trouble shooting with the patient, relaying outcomes and treatment needs or problems to the psychiatrist, and keeping the PCP well informed of any treatment or medication changes or recommendations. Use of a standardized form, which may be hard copy or, ideally, electronic, creates a continuous record of the patient's course, tracking symptoms (repeated administrations of the Patient Health Questionnaire-9 [PHQ-9[58]], a 10-item self-administered tool that quantifies the severity of depression-related symptoms), medication trials (eg, reporting drug, dose, adjustment, side effects, augmentation), other modalities (eg, talk therapy), treatment adherence, and other issues (eg, psychosocial events, other medical issues). In more recent years, the model has been expanded to treat posttraumatic stress disorder in military cohorts. With some work to replace the PHQ-9 with other severity measures, the general tenets of the model could be adapted for evidence-based treatment of a wider range of primary care mental health issues.

PRIMARY CARE–DRIVEN MODEL

A pragmatic primary care–driven model,[59] derived with the sole purpose to meet the demands of primary care management of mental health issues in a large, inner city, immigrant community health center, fluidly incorporates features of collaborative management, TCM, and other models (eg, teleconsultation). Ideally, the psychiatrist is a member of the clinic medical staff, but could also be a well-known, consistent consultant who works closely with the clinic physicians and other staff. The goal of the model is to provide high-quality, cost-effective treatment within the clinic for patients whose mental health issues can be managed by their PCPs, and to assist with appropriate referral for quality community-based care, as necessary. The scope of the model is not diagnostically determined (eg, treatment of depression or anxiety); rather, the main consideration is whether the patient's problems are likely to be manageable by the PCP. An assumption of this model is that some patients (eg, patients who are suicidal, homicidal, or severely character-disordered) and some disorders (eg, psychotic, bipolar, or primary addictive disorders) are not sufficiently stable for ongoing treatment in primary care. Therefore, the model requires the availability of adequate community services for the referral of such patients.

Referrals come from the PCP, the broker of all specialty care. The psychiatrist has a flexible array of service offerings from curbside consultation (in person), telephone consultation, shared visits (in which the psychiatrist is invited into to the PCP's visit with the patient), or formal scheduled evaluations. Even with a limited resource (eg, a single, perhaps part-time, psychiatrist), access can be exceptional because of this variety of real-time services and the PCPs knowledge of, and rapport with, the patient. The PCP may be willing to start treatment with input from the known psychiatric consultant. If the psychiatrist schedules an appointment to evaluate the patient, the patient is not losing time untreated and the psychiatrist has more data by the time of the evaluation. Some patients who are afraid to see a psychiatrist can be introduced to one in the safety of their PCP's office and presence, opening the door to future visits if necessary. If the psychiatrist does a formal evaluation of the patient and starts treatment, the goal is to see the patient several times as necessary to establish improvement and sufficient stability for PCP management. The patient must be adequately, and sometimes repeatedly, informed of the intent to return their care to the PCP. This decreases the possible sense of rejection, when the PCP refers the patient for a consultation, or abandonment, when the psychiatrist returns the patient, with ongoing recommendations, to the PCP's care. If the patient experiences worsening symptoms during previously effective treatment (roughening), or other medical and/ or social stressors destabilize them, they may again see the, now familiar, psychiatrist for a brief period of treatment. Because the psychiatrist is within the circle of care, there may be a single medical record, and the intent to communicate must be made clear to the patient.

This model is most effective when coupled with in-house masters-level clinicians who provide focused, goal-oriented, brief, culturally sensitive, individual or group talk therapies in the patient's primary language. When patients require referral, those with more complicated issues, requiring multiple provider or agency involvement, benefit from collaborative care management to broker fragmented services into a coordinated network of care, with signed releases and facilitated communication back to the PCP.

An excellent opportunity to train the next generation of collaborative psychiatrists and PCPs (a resident physician training site), this model requires ongoing education, formal and informal, to improve both the internal capacity for quality treatment and recognition of those issues that require specialist care.

SUMMARY

Although changes in the US health care system promote a population-based approach, increases in population diversity emphasize the need for culturally competent, patient-centered, participatory care. Despite this perceived conflict, the global view has improved the recognition of mental health issues as a driver of overall health, as well as health care spending. This recognition, along with the many forces that keep mental health care in the primary care sector, actually encourages the development of collaborative models that capitalize on the PCP's opportunity to leverage their rapport with the patient to improve access to, and comfort with, specialty mental health services. For full effectiveness of any of these models, all parties must be actively and continuously educated, all treating clinicians should strive for cultural competence or humility, physicians (primary care and specialist) should listen and appreciate that patient is the expert on all aspects of their own cultural identity and beliefs. Engaging the patient in their own path to recovery or well-being improves engagement in, and adherence to, the treatment plan, and ultimately improves outcomes.

REFERENCES

1. McKegney FP. After a century of C-L psychiatry, whither goest C-L in the 21st? [abstract]. Psychosomatics 1995;36:202–3.

2. Committee on Quality Health Care in America, Institute of Medicine. Crossing the quality chasm: a new health system for the 21st century. Washington, DC: National Academy Press; 2001.

3. The introduction of chlorpromazine. Hosp Community Psychiatry 1976;27:505.

4. Regier DA, Narrow WE, Rae DS, et al. The de facto US mental and addictive disorders system. Arch Gen Psychiatry 1993;50:85–94.

5. Kessler RC, Berglund P, Demler O, et al. The epidemiology of major depressive disorder, results from the National Comorbidity Survey Replication (NCS-R). JAMA 2003;289:3095–105.

6. Eisenberg L. Treating depression and anxiety in primary care: closing the gap between knowledge and practice. N Engl J Med 1992;326:1080–4.

7. Shapiro S, German PS, Skinner EA, et al. An experiment to change detection and management of mental morbidity in primary care. Med Care 1987;25:327–39.

8. Tiemens BG, Ormel J, Simon GE. Occurrence, recognition, and outcome of psychological disorders in primary care. Am J Psychiatry 1996;153:636–44.

9. Barrett JE, Barrett JA, Oxman TE, et al. The prevalence of psychiatric disorders in a primary care practice. Arch Gen Psychiatry 1988;45:1100–6.

10. Coyne JC, Schwenk TL, Fechner-Bates S. Nondetection of depression by primary care physicians reconsidered. Gen Hosp Psychiatry 1995;17:3–12.

11. Roy-Byrne PP, Katon W, Cowley DS, et al. Panic disorder in primary care: biopsychosocial differences between recognized and unrecognized patients. Gen Hosp Psychiatry 2000;22:405–11.

12. Wang PS, Demler O, Olfson M, et al. Changing profiles of service sectors used for mental health care in the United States. Am J Psychiatry 2006;163:1187–98.

13. Unützer J, Schoenbaum M, Druss BG, et al. Transforming metal health care at the interface with general medicine: report for the President's Commission. Psychiatr Serv 2006;57:37–47.

14. Vanderpool HK, de Bittner MR, Cuellar L, et al. Report of the ASHP Ad Hoc Committee on ethnic diversity and cultural competence. Am J Health Syst Pharm 2005;62:1924–30.

15. Cooper LA, Gonzales JJ, Gallo JJ, et al. The acceptability of treatment for depression among African-American, Hispanic, and white primary care patients. Med Care 2003;31:479–89.

16. Nadeem E, Lange JM, Edge D, et al. Does stigma keep poor young immigrant and U.S.-born black and Latina women from seeking mental health care? Psychiatr Serv 2007;58:1547–54.

17. Johnson J, Weissman MM, Klerman GL. Service utilization and social morbidity associated with depressive symptoms in the community. JAMA 1992;267:1478–83.

18. Simon GE, Khandker RK, Ichikawa L, et al. Recovery from depression predicts lower health service costs. J Clin Psychiatry 2006;67:1226–31.

19. Stewart WF, Ricci JA, Chee E, et al. Cost of lost productive work time among US workers with depression. JAMA 2003;289:3135–44.

20. Broadhead WE, Blazer DG, George LK, et al. Depression, disability days, and days lost from work in a prospective epidemiological study. JAMA 1990;264:2524–8.

21. Bendapudi NM, Berry LL, Frey KA, et al. Patients' perspectives on ideal physician behaviors. Mayo Clin Proc 2006;81:338–44.

22. Beach MC, Sugarman J, Johnson RL, et al. Do patients treated with dignity report higher satisfaction, adherence, and receipt of preventive care? Ann Fam Med 2005;3:331–8.

23. Platt FW, Gaspar DL, Coulehan JL, et al. The patient-centered interview. Ann Intern Med 2001;134:1079–85.

24. Carrillo JE, Green AR, Betancourt JR. Cross-cultural primary care: a patient-based approach. Ann Intern Med 1999;130:829–34.
25. Beck RS, Daughtridge R, Sloane PD. Physician-patient communication in the primary care office: a systematic review. J Am Board Fam Pract 2002;15:25–38.
26. Weiner SJ, Barnet B, Cheng TL, et al. Processes for effective communication in primary care. Ann Intern Med 2005;142:709–14.
27. Safran DG. Defining the future of primary care: what can we learn from patients? Ann Intern Med 2003;138:248–55.
28. Gordon C, Beresin EV. The doctor-patient relationship. In: Stern TA, Rosenbaum JF, Fava M, et al, editors. Massachusetts General Hospital comprehensive clinical psychiatry. Philadelphia: Mosby; 2008. p. 13–26.
29. Tervalon M, Murray-Garcia J. Cultural humility versus cultural competence: a critical distinction in defining physician training outcomes in multicultural education. J Health Care Poor Underserved 1998;9:117–25.
30. Van Orden M, Hoffman T, Haffmans J, et al. Collaborative mental health care versus care a usual in primary care setting: a randomized controlled trial. Psychiatr Serv 2009;60:74–9.
31. Beresin EV, Gordon C. The psychiatric interview. In: Stern TA, Rosenbaum JF, Fava M, et al, editors. Massachusetts General Hospital comprehensive clinical psychiatry. Philadelphia: Mosby; 2008. p. 27–49.
32. Pinderhughes E. Understanding race, ethnicity and power: the key to efficacy in clinical practice. New York: Free Press; 1989.
33. Fox RC. Cultural competence and the culture of medicine. N Engl J Med 2005;353:1316–9.
34. Marvel MK, Epstein RM, Flowers K, et al. Soliciting the patient's agenda: have we improved? JAMA 1999;281:283–7.
35. Charon R. Narrative medicine: a model for empathy, reflection, profession and trust. JAMA 2001;286:1897–902.
36. Gordon C, Goroll A. Effective psychiatric interviewing in primary care medicine. In: Stern TA, Herman JB, Slavin PL, editors. The MGH guide to primary care psychiatry. New York: McGraw-Hill; 2004. p. 19–27.
37. Hak T, Campion P. Achieving a patient-centered consultation by giving feedback in its early stages. Postgrad Med J 1999;75:405–9.
38. Haidet P, Paterniti DA. "Building" a history rather than "taking" one: a perspective on information sharing during the interview. Arch Intern Med 2003;163:1134–40.
39. Lazare A. Shame and humiliation in the medical encounter. Arch Intern Med 1987;147:1653–8.
40. Fischer D, Stewart AL, Bloch DA, et al. Capturing the patient's view of change as a clinical outcome measure. JAMA 1999;282:1157–62.
41. Cooper-Patrick L, Gallo JJ, Gonzales JJ, et al. Race, gender, and partnerships in the patient-physician relationship. JAMA 1999;282:583–9.
42. Betancourt JR, Alexander RG, Carrillo JE. Cultural competence in health care: emerging frameworks and practical approaches. Washington, DC: The Commonwealth Fund; 2002.
43. O'Connor PJ. Improving medication adherence: challenges for physicians, payers, and policy makers. Arch Intern Med 2006;166:1802–4.
44. Haynes RB, McDonald HP, Garg AX. Helping patients follow prescribed treatment. JAMA 2002;288:2880–3.
45. Stewart M, Brown JB, Donner A, et al. The impact of patient-centered care on outcomes. J Fam Pract 2000;49:796–804.

46. Levinson W, Gorawara-Bhat R, Dueck R, et al. Resolving disagreements in the patient-physician relationship. JAMA 1999;282:1477–83.
47. Stevenson FA, Barry CA, Britten N, et al. Doctor-patient communication about drugs: the evidence for shared decision making. Soc Sci Med 2000;50:829–40.
48. Deegan PE, Drake RE. Shared decision making and medication management in the recovery process. Psychiatr Serv 2006;57:1636–8.
49. Katon W, Von Korff M, Lin E, et al. Collaborative management to achieve treatment guidelines: impact on depression in primary care. JAMA 1995;273:1026–31.
50. Robinson P. Integrated treatment of depression in primary care. Strategic Medicine 1997;1:22–9.
51. Katon WJ, Schoenbaum M, Fan M-Y, et al. Cost-effectiveness of improving primary care treatment of late-life depression. Arch Gen Psychiatry 2005;62:1313–20.
52. Katon W, Von Korff M, Lin E, et al. Stepped collaborative care for primary care patients with persistent symptoms of depression. Arch Gen Psychiatry 1999;56:1109–15.
53. Unutzer J, Katon W, Callahan CM, et al. Collaborative care management of late-life depression in the primary care setting, a randomized controlled trial. JAMA 2002;288:2836–45.
54. Druss BG, Rohrbaugh RM, Levinson CM, et al. Integrated medical care for patients with serious psychiatric illness. Arch Gen Psychiatry 2001;58:861–8.
55. Beck BJ. Approaches to collaborative care and primary care psychiatry. In: Stern TA, Rosenbaum JF, Fava M, et al, editors. Massachusetts General Hospital comprehensive clinical psychiatry. Philadelphia: Mosby; 2008. p. 811–9.
56. Katon WJ, Roy-Byrne P, Russo J, et al. Cost-effectiveness and cost offset of a collaborative care intervention for primary care patients with panic disorder. Arch Gen Psychiatry 2002;59:1098–104.
57. Oxman T, Dietrich AJ, Williams JW, et al. A three-component model for reengineering systems for the treatment of depression in primary care. Psychosomatics 2002;43:441–50.
58. Kroenke K, Spitzer RL. The PHQ-9: a new depression diagnostic and severity measure. Psychiatr Ann 2002;32:509–616.
59. Pirl WF, Beck BJ, Safren SA, et al. A descriptive study of psychiatric consultations in a community primary care center. Prim Care Companion J Clin Psychiatry 2001;3:190–4.

An Approach to the Patient in Crisis: Assessments of the Risk of Suicide and Violence

Rebecca Weintraub Brendel, MD, JD[a,b,*],
Marlynn H. Wei, MD, JD[a,b], Judith G. Edersheim, JD, MD[a,b]

KEYWORDS

- Suicidal ideation - Psychiatric disorder - Violence
- Personality disorder

Patients in crisis and in jeopardy of harming themselves, others, or both are seen by their physicians. The internist is in an excellent position to intervene with patients at risk for suicide in light of the understanding that most patients who commit suicide have seen their primary care physicians (PCPs) in the year before their death[1] and nearly 50% of patients have had contact with their PCP in the month preceding their suicide.[1–3] Management of patients in crisis is often anxiety-provoking for clinicians and may even lead clinicians to wonder if they can do anything at all to help the patient. This article outlines the elements of the risk assessment (for harm to self and/or others) and addresses which contributing factors may be modifiable. This article also proposes a practical framework for the management of risk regarding suicide and violence.

SUICIDE

Suicide, the 11th leading cause of death in the United States, is defined as intentional self-harm with the intent of causing death.[4] Self-inflicted injuries account for nearly 600,000 (0.5%) emergency department visits and approximately 33,000 deaths in the United States each year.[4,5]

[a] Department of Psychiatry, Massachusetts General Hospital, 15 Parkman Street, WAC 812, Boston, MA 02114, USA
[b] Department of Psychiatry, Harvard Medical School, 25 Shattuck Street, Boston, MA 02115, USA
* Corresponding author. Department of Psychiatry, Massachusetts General Hospital, 15 Parkman Street, WAC 812, Boston, MA 02114.
E-mail address: rbrendel@partners.org

Med Clin N Am 94 (2010) 1089–1102
doi:10.1016/j.mcna.2010.08.002
0025-7125/10/$ – see front matter © 2010 Elsevier Inc. All rights reserved.

medical.theclinics.com

Although psychiatric disorders are associated with more than 90% of completed suicides,[6,7] individuals with medical illness, especially of a severe or chronic nature, are at an increased risk of suicide.[8–10] Medical disorders are noted in as many as one-third to 40% of suicides; as many as 70% of suicides occur in those older than 60 years.[11,12]

Knowledge of risk factors for suicide can help in identifying patients at a heightened risk for suicide. One study found that the use of the Geriatric Depression Scale successfully identified older patients with suicidal ideation.[13,14] However, because suicide is uncommon, testing positive during screening for risk factors should be followed by a more thorough risk assessment. Using trained care managers within physician practices has been shown to decrease suicidal ideation and to achieve remission of major depression.[15]

Epidemiology and Risk Factors

Suicide accounts for approximately 1% of all deaths in the United States.[16,17] For every completed suicide, approximately 8 to 10 individuals attempt suicide and between 8 and 25 attempts are made.[18–22] The most common method of completed suicide involves the use of firearms; suffocation and poisoning are also frequently used methods.[4] Drug ingestion is the method most commonly used in unsuccessful suicide attempts.[23,24] Suicide rates increase with advancing age, with individuals older than 65 years being 1.5 times more likely to commit suicide than younger individuals; men older than 85 years are at an even higher risk.[25–27] Men more frequently complete suicide than do women, but women attempt suicide more frequently.[17,28,29]

The most powerful risk factor for suicide, present in more than 90% of completed suicides, is the presence of mental illness.[6,7,28,30] Among psychiatric disorders, mood disorders (eg, major depression and bipolar disorder) are found in approximately half of completed suicides; this represents a 30-fold greater risk of suicide than those in the general population.[31–34] Substance abuse disorders are evident in roughly one-fourth of completed suicides, psychosis is present in 10%, and personality disorders are noted in 5%.[31,32] Therefore, a history of mental illness should alert the internist to the potential for a patient's self-harm. In addition, suicide attempts are noted in half of those who eventually commit suicide, and the risk for completed suicide in the year after an unsuccessful attempt is estimated at nearly 100 times the risk of those in the general population.[21,35,36]

Medical illness itself is associated with a higher risk of suicide and occurs in 35% to 40% of completed suicides and in as many as 70% of suicides in patients older than 60 years.[8–12] Suicide is more common in patients with AIDS, cancer, traumatic brain injury, epilepsy, multiple sclerosis, Huntington disease, organic brain syndromes, spinal cord injuries, hypertension, cardiopulmonary disease, peptic ulcer disease, chronic renal failure, Cushing disease, rheumatoid arthritis, and porphyria.[37] Severe or chronic illness predisposes to an increased suicide risk.[37] Among patients with chronic illnesses, those with renal failure on hemodialysis may be at the highest risk (as high as 400 times that of the general population).[38] Patients with human immunodeficiency virus infection seem to be 7 to 66 times more likely to commit suicide than those in the general population.[31,39,40] Other illnesses are associated with a 2- to 5-fold increase in the rate of suicide over that of the general population.[37]

A history of suicide in a family member, likely mediated primarily through genetic factors, although shared family environments in which modeling and imitation occur are also seen as contributing factors[36,41–43] doubles the risk of suicide, even after controlling for psychiatric diagnoses.[44] Social risk factors (eg, being widowed, divorced, or separated; living alone; and being socially isolated) are associated with an increased risk of suicide.[2,11,41,45,46] Significant personal losses and conflicts (eg, bereavement, unemployment, and financial and legal difficulties) have also been identified as risk factors.[6,11,12,21,36,47–49] Presence of a firearm in the home also seems to be an independent risk factor for suicide for both genders.[47,50,51]

Clinical Presentation and Evaluation

Patients at risk of suicide have varied presentations (eg, have unexpressed wishes to be dead or may be critically ill following a near-lethal suicide attempt). Evaluation of such patients requires a comprehensive assessment, beginning with an assessment of risk factors. However, risk factors alone do not predict the risk of suicide and are neither sensitive nor specific.[37,52,53] Instead, patients at an increased risk of suicide should have a thorough psychiatric examination.

Practice guidelines support an assessment approach that includes interrogation specifically about thoughts of suicide and plans to commit suicide, examination of the details of a suicide plan, determination of a risk to rescue ratio, assessment of the level of planning and preparation, evaluation of the degree of hopelessness, and identification of precipitants. A multiaxial psychiatric diagnosis should be made, and the risk of suicide estimated.[54] Consultation with other providers, past and present, is generally helpful in understanding a patient's current level of suicidal ideation. Interview of family, friends, and other third parties can corroborate clinical information obtained from the patient.[21,48,55] Overall, the approach to a patient who may be at risk for suicide should be supportive, empathic, and nonjudgmental; efforts should be taken to maximize the privacy and physical comfort of the interview setting.[55]

Evaluation of the suicidal patient centers on an open and direct approach to key features associated with suicide risk. Clinicians may worry about offending a patient by asking direct questions about suicidality. However, patients are often relieved when they encounter someone with whom they can speak openly about troubling thoughts; there is no evidence that nonsuicidal patients become suicidal by virtue of direct questioning about suicidal ideation.[41,55,56] Effective interviewing of a potentially suicidal patient flows from general, open-ended questions about thoughts of hopelessness and/or loss of desire to live to more specific questions about suicidal thoughts and plans for suicide.[41,55,57] For example, an organized and detailed plan with a readily available and highly lethal means is generally more concerning to clinicians than is the presence of passive thoughts of death without an identified plan or means. Clinicians often calculate a risk to rescue ratio of suicide attempts; the greater the potential lethality of an attempt and the lower the risk of rescue, the more serious the suicide risk.[54,58] Patients should be asked directly about plans and hopes for the future, because hopelessness and a lack of future plans are associated with a higher risk of suicide.[55]

Management of Suicide Risk

The first step in the treatment of suicide risk involves stabilization of the medical sequelae of self-injurious behaviors. If the suicidal patient is being medically stabilized or if the patient is suicidal but has not yet acted on suicidal thoughts, a safe environment must be provided for the patient. A treatment plan for the suicidal patient requires the maintenance of safety, determination of the appropriate setting for treatment, development of a medical plan for pharmacologic or somatic therapy intervention, frequent reassessment of safety and suicide risk, and measurement of treatment response. Potential means for self-harm (eg, open windows, available means of egress, and sharp objects) should be blocked or removed. Although the least restrictive, but effective, method of ensuring safety should be invoked, one-to-one supervision may be necessary, and for high-risk patients who have made serious attempts or who cannot control their suicidal impulses, hospitalization on a locked unit may be required. Practitioners should become aware of the legal and regulatory requirements in the jurisdictions in which they practice (regarding involuntary evaluation, holding, and/or treatment of suicidal patients). When uncertainty lingers regarding the patient's risk, clinicians should err on the side of caution and protect the patient.[55] Although frequently used, safety contracts (between patients and providers) have never been shown to be effective.[54,59] Psychiatric consultation may be obtained to provide the suicide risk assessment and facilitate transfer to the most appropriate treatment setting.

The patient should be fully evaluated to establish a multiaxial psychiatric diagnosis. Once underlying psychiatric conditions and other associated stressors or circumstances are identified, a treatment plan (combining medications, therapies, and/or other interventions) can be developed and the patient's progress assessed on an ongoing basis.[37] Because depression is the diagnosis most clearly associated with suicide, antidepressants are often a mainstay of psychiatric treatment of the suicidal patient. It is important for clinicians to be aware that all the medications in the selective serotonin reuptake inhibitor (SSRI) class have black box warnings regarding their potential to increase suicidal thoughts. Nonetheless, because of their favorable side-effect profile and safety in overdose (compared with tricyclic antidepressants and monoamine oxidase inhibitors), SSRIs remain the first-line treatment for the depressed, suicidal patient. Electroconvulsive therapy also leads to rapid remission of mood disorders. Among pharmacologic interventions, long-term lithium treatment in affective illness and clozapine in schizophrenia have been shown to reduce the risk of suicide.[60–63]

Clinicians should be aware of their potential for strong reactions (eg, anger, anxiety, helplessness, rejection, denial, intellectualization, depression, indifference, and over-identification with the patient) to suicidal patients or to those who have attempted suicide[64] and should be on guard so as not to have them interfere with the assessment, stabilization, and treatment of suicidal patients. Highly charged situations should be dealt with and diffused so that the emotions of staff do not interfere with the patient's best interests.[65]

VIOLENCE TO OTHERS

PCPs must also assess a patient's potential for violence in a variety of settings.[66] This is no easy task, as violence is a multifactorial and complex behavior, with social, psychological, and biologic determinants.[67] Any attempt to assess future dangerousness in an individual should be undertaken with caution, as the current state of risk assessment is fraught with statistical and methodological errors and limitations inherent in applying the epidemiologic risk factors to low base rate phenomena.[68] When assessing the potential for future violence, one should consider some threshold characteristics of violence; the leading risk factors for violence are youth, male gender, low socioeconomic status, and a history of violence.[69] Some threatened or actual violence is mediated by mental illness, and therefore, every clinician should have an approach to patients who are aggressive or violent during a clinical encounter.[70,71]

The Link Between Violence and Mental Illness

For the past 50 years, researchers have tried to elucidate the complex and intricate link between violence and mental disorders.[72] Although this body of research is vast, serious violent behavior is uncommon among persons with mental disorders and most violent acts have no relationship to mental illness. However, certain psychiatric illnesses are associated with a modest increase in the risk of future violence.[73,74] Even in studies that have attempted to isolate subsets of patients with severe mental illness to identify a high point for this number, the prevalence of serious assaultive behaviors in this cohort remains low.[75–77] Most of the research on the association between violence and mental illness establishes correlations between past violence and lifetime psychiatric diagnoses rather than establishing mental illness as an independent risk factor for violent behavior.[74] It seems that the increase in violence among subsets of patients who are mentally ill has a complex and incompletely understood relationship with coexisting demographic, contextual, and clinical factors.

Psychiatric disorders
The prevalence rates of violent behavior in patients with mental illness is on the order of 3 to 5 times greater than in patients without mental illness, with different levels of increased risk associated with personality disorders, mood disorders, and thought disorders.[78] However, this absolute number remains small in light of the low base rate of violence in the community.[78] Substance abuse disorders increase the risk of violence to a far greater extent than any other mental illness, and some diagnostic categories present a higher risk than others.

Substance abuse disorders
It has become increasingly apparent that substance abuse is a highly significant risk factor for future violence, whether alone or in combination with other mental disorders.[79,80] Adults with substance abuse disorders are approximately 12 to 16 times more likely than adults without a substance abuse history to commit a violent act, and active substance abuse has an additive effect in increasing the risk in persons with major mental disorders.[75] Some researchers of risk assessment have asserted that when substance abuse is controlled for, the prevalence of violence among patients who are mentally ill matches the rate for community controls.[79] In contrast, others contend that not all of the increased risk is because of substance abuse but is accounted for by other diagnoses (eg, conduct disorders or psychosis).[74] Regardless of the outcome of this debate, the presence of an active substance abuse disorder disproportionately increases the risk for future violence and is a critical area in which screening by PCPs may be effective.

Personality disorders
Personality disorders (particularly antisocial, borderline, and narcissistic personality disorders) are associated with a higher risk for violent behavior.[81] Among those conditions, antisocial personality disorder and its analogue in the psychology literature, psychopathy, seem to be robust predictors of aggressive behavior,[82] particularly in the context of criminal recidivism.[83] These 3 disorders are often comorbid with substance abuse, and in combination, they place a patient into a higher-risk category when assessing the potential for violence. The association between psychopathy and the risk for future violence is so robust that specific diagnostic assessment tools for this disorder are commonly used as screening tools in correctional settings for the determination of detention services and parole.[84,85]

Psychotic disorders
Research on the relationship between psychotic disorders and the risk of violence is conflicting and confusing. Studies from the 1990s consistently showed a significant correlation between patients with thought disorders and both inpatient and outpatient violence.[86] Specifically, persecutory delusions,[87] command hallucinations[88] (to harm

others), and so-called threat/control/override symptoms[89] were identified as reliable indicators of an increased likelihood of future violence. However, during the past 10 years, several studies have challenged this notion, concluding that persecutory or threat/control/override symptoms are unrelated to violence; these effects are the result of character traits (eg, suspiciousness, anger, impulsivity).[90] Others have found that delusions may actually decrease the risk of violence.[91] One way to understand these divergent data is to separate the effects of the so-called positive symptoms of psychosis or schizophrenia (eg, delusions, hallucinations, persecutory hostility) that intuitively might increase the propensity for a violent response from effects of the negative symptoms (eg, apathy, social withdrawal, passivity) that might make a coordinated violent response less likely.[92] Pending a conclusive resolution of these conflicting data, it is prudent to consider active psychotic symptoms as an indicator of an increased potential for violence.[92]

Social and Demographic Factors

Social and demographic factors are more likely than mental illness to contribute to violence risk.[78] An awareness of these risk factors is necessary during clinical risk assessments, and these factors should be considered when attempting to intervene or ameliorate risk.

Youth, male gender, and low socioeconomic status are some of the leading demographic risk factors for violence.[75] Among all risk factors, history of violence is the best predictor.[68] Clinicians should explore the nature and severity of prior violence and the age at which it occurred because early violence, early conduct problems, early arrest, and juvenile detention are historical features that correlate with an increase in the risk for subsequent violent acts.[93] Antisocial traits (eg, parental criminal history, parental substance abuse, parental physical abuse) in one or both parents also increase risk.[74] The nature of interfamilial interactions also influences the propensity for aggressive behavior. Children raised in families that manifest, condone, or encourage violence as a solution to daily problems are at an increased risk for perpetuating violent responses.[94]

Violence occurs in a social context and is influenced by internal and external factors, which can either exacerbate or decrease risk.[95] In general, patients who report a high degree of stress, particularly in the context of poor social support, are at a higher risk for future aggression.[93] Specific major life stressors (eg, job loss, homelessness, loss of loved ones [whether through death, divorce, or separation]) seem to increase the risk for aggressive behavior. A history of personal victimization and the nature and age at the time of such victimization have also been associated with the risk of future violence.[78] Of particular concern is the patient with a history of violence who is presenting in a similar context, with an available victim and an available means of harm or attack.[93] Studies have also demonstrated an association between firearm ownership and both suicide and homicide.[96] In contrast, the presence of protective factors (eg, religious or spiritual beliefs, a capacity for empathy, social efficacy, and respect) might place someone in a lower-risk category.[95]

Clinical Traits

A myriad of clinical variables have been linked to an increase in the risk of future violence and can be grouped under diagnostic considerations and clinical status.[69] With respect to diagnostic considerations, the diagnosis of a mental illness modestly increases the lifetime risk of committing a violent act; this risk is significantly increased when combined with substance abuse. However, these diagnoses rarely occur in isolation, and several attributes are often related to this increased risk. Neurologic impairment and cognitive deficits increase the risk of future violence, most likely because these impairments can increase impulsivity, decrease frustration tolerance, and deprive individuals of the cognitive flexibility that provides alternatives to violent responses.[97] Certain affective tendencies, regardless of diagnosis, enhance the propensity for violence. Hypervigilance, impulsivity, anger, a hostile attributional bias, and poor affect regulation have each been identified as personality traits that make violent responses more likely.[98,99] With respect to clinical status, patients who are not engaged in their mental health treatment or who are noncompliant with medications present an increased risk for violence.[100] Patients who believe that they need treatment and that their treatment has been effective are significantly less likely to commit a violent act.[101]

RISK ASSESSMENT SKILLS

Several strategies are available for the assessment of the risk of future violent behavior, and these strategies vary by methodology and treatment population. Typically, the methodology selected is based on the setting (eg, emergency service, inpatient, outpatient, forensic), the goal (eg, triage, treatment, discharge planning, disposition), and the amount of information that is available to the clinician regarding the patient (eg, patient interviews, extensive demographic information).

In forensic and correctional settings, clinicians often use actuarial instruments for risk assessment, sometimes in combination with clinical or dynamic risk formulations. These actuarial instruments estimate risk categories by tabulating static or historical risk information about the patient to assign a risk level relative to other people. The Hare Psychopathy Checklist[102] and the Violence Risk Appraisal Guide[103] are just 2 examples of well-established actuarial instruments; others are tailored to specific populations and used in different clinical contexts.[104] Although these instruments offer great statistical accuracy and are useful with heterogeneous populations, they are insensitive to individual variations in risk; they do not take into account changes associated with treatment or other contextual modifications.[73] Although many offer shorter screening versions of the full actuarial assessment,[105] clinicians often do not have access to the large amount of clinical and historical data required for scoring these instruments.

Most physicians use unaided clinical predictions to estimate violence risk; however, this method is statistically inferior to actuarial assessments or to a combination of actuarial and clinical risk factors.[106] When performing such unstructured clinical risk assessments, evaluators tend to overestimate the risk of violence, overemphasize treatable variables (eg, medication compliance), and underestimate social and environmental variables,[107] which result in low interrater reliability and a poor positive predictive value.[108] However, clinical assessment tends to be more accurate in inpatient settings than in outpatient settings, leading some to suggest that static risk factors may be best for evaluating long-term violence risk and clinical factors, for the evaluation of imminent risk in acutely ill patients.[109]

The preferred method for risk evaluation in the clinical setting is to use a combination approach or a fusion of empirically validated risk factors informed by clinical data to come up with an estimation of the level of risk.[110] Several instruments offer this structured professional judgment (eg, the Historical, Clinical, and Risk Management [HCR]-20,[111] the Classification of Violence Risk,[112] and the Iterative Classification Tree[76]). These instruments tend to be more relevant to clinical populations, and they incorporate clinical judgment and treatment variables. The HCR is the best known of these scales, with 10 historical variables and 5 clinical variables, as well as 5 risk management variables that address contextual destabilizers and barriers to treatment.

Box 1
Factors associated with increased risk of violence

Diagnostic factors

Substance abuse

Psychopathy/antisocial personality disorder

Active psychotic symptoms

Major mental disorder

Demographic factors

Youth (age 15 to 24 years)

Male gender

Low socioeconomic status

Low educational level

Historical factors

History of violence or criminality

Early age at first offense

History of conduct difficulties

Violence or abuse in family

History of parental criminality

Family modeling of violence

History of parental criminality

Contextual factors

Perceived stress

Poor social support

Availability of victims

Availability of weapons or means

Similar context to previous violence

Current use of alcohol/stimulants

Social factors

Recent death, loss, separation

Unemployment/job loss

Homelessness/residential instability

Clinical/affective traits

Neurologic impairment

Cognitive deficits

Impulsivity

Anger

Hypervigilance

Hostile attributional bias

Data from Borum R, Swartz M, Swanson J. Assessing and managing violence risk in clinical practice. J Prac Psych Behav Health 1996;4:205–15.

The Future of Risk Assessment for Violent Behavior

The assessment of an individual's risk for future violence involves attention to a myriad of interrelated risk factors, including clinical, historical, demographic, contextual, and social variables (**Box 1**). The past 50 years of risk assessment research has resulted in an improved set of variables associated with violence, although the causal mechanisms linking these variables with aggression are not completely understood. Future risk assessment research will, out of necessity, involve refining these variables and elucidating their causal nexus to violent behavior; it will also involve translating these risk assessment data into strategies for risk management and risk reduction. There will be a focus on methods to intervene with clinically modifiable risk factors, whether through treatment or through extended wraparound community services. Clinicians will need to use improved techniques to monitor intraindividual variations in the level of risk.[113]

REFERENCES

1. Luoma JB, Martin CE, Pearson JL. Contact with mental health and primary care providers before suicide: a review of the evidence. Am J Psychiatry 2002;159: 909–16.
2. Hirschfeld RM. Algorithm for the evaluation and treatment of suicidal patients. Prim Psychiatry 1996;3:26–9.
3. Fawcett J, Clark DC, Busch KA. Assessing and treating the patient at risk for suicide. Psychiatr Ann 1993;23:244–55.
4. Centers for Disease Control and Prevention. Suicide and self-inflicted injury. 2006. Available at: http://www.cdc.gov/nchs/fastats/suicide.htm. Accessed June 13, 2010.
5. U.S. Department of health and human services national health statistics report 12008, no 7. 2008. Available at: http://www.cdc.gov/nchs/data/nhsr/nhsr007.pdf. Accessed June 13, 2010.
6. Rich CL, Young D, Fowler RC. San Diego suicide study: young vs old subjects. Arch Gen Psychiatry 1986;43:577–82.
7. Brent DA. Correlates of medical lethality of suicide attempts in children and adolescents. J Am Acad Child Adolesc Psychiatry 1987;26:87–9.
8. Maris RW. Suicide. Lancet 2002;360:319–26.
9. Silverman MM, Goldblatt MJ. Physical illness and suicide. In: Maris RW, Berman AL, Silverman MM, editors. Comprehensive textbook of suicidology. New York: Guilford Press; 2000. p. 342–56.
10. Hughes K, Kleepies P. Suicide in the medically ill. Suicide Life Threat Behav 2001;(Suppl):48–60.
11. Maris RW. Suicide and life-threatening behavior. Introduction. Suicide Life Threat Behav 1991;21:1–17.
12. Conwell Y, Duberstein PR. Suicide among older people: a problem for primary care. Prim Psychiatry 1996;3:41–4.
13. Heisel MJ, Duberstein PR, Lyness JM, et al. Screening for suicide ideation among older primary care patients. J Am Board Fam Med 2010;23:260–9.
14. Hegerl U, Wittenburg L, Arensman E, et al. Optimizing suicide prevention programs and their implementation in Europe (OSPI Europe): an evidence-based multi-level approach. BMC Public Health 2009;9:428.
15. Alexopoulos GS, Reynolds CF, Bruce ML, et al. Reducing suicidal ideation and depression in older primary care patients: 24-month outcomes of the PROSPECT study. Am J Psychiatry 2009;166:882–90.

16. Kochanek KD, Murphy SL, Anderson RN, et al. Deaths: final data for 2002. Natl Vital Stat Rep 2004;53(5):1–116.

17. Moscicki E. Epidemiology of suicide. In: Goldsmith S, editor. Risk factors for suicide. Washington, DC: National Academy Press; 2001. p. 1–3.

18. Clayton PJ. Suicide. Psychiatr Clin North Am 1985;8:203–14.

19. Hirschfeld RM, Davidson L. Risk factors for suicide. In: Frances AJ, Hales RE, editors. American psychiatric press review of psychiatry, vol. 7. Washington, DC: American Psychiatric Press; 1988.

20. Malone KM, Haas GL, Sweeney JA, et al. Major depression and the risk of attempted suicide. J Affect Disord 1995;34:173–85.

21. Moscicki EK. Epidemiology of suicidal behavior. Suicide Life Threat Behav 1995; 2:22–35.

22. National Institute of Mental Health. Suicide facts and statistics. Available at: http://www.nimh.nih.gov/health/publications/suicide-in-the-us-statistics-and-prevention/index.shtml. Accessed June 26, 2010.

23. Weissman MM. The epidemiology of suicide attempts, 1960–1971. Arch Gen Psychiatry 1974;30:737–46.

24. Andrus JK, Fleming DW, Heumann MA, et al. Surveillance of attempted suicide among adolescents in Oregon, 1988. Am J Public Health 1991;81:1067–9.

25. Gaynes BN, West SL, Ford CA, et al. Screening for suicide risk in adults: a summary of the evidence for the U.S. Preventive Services Task Force. Ann Intern Med 2004;140:822–35.

26. McIntosh JL. Suicide prevention in the elderly (age 65–99). Suicide Life Threat Behav 1995;25:180–92.

27. O'Connell H, Chin A, Cunningham C, et al. Recent developments: suicide in older people. BMJ 2004;329:895–9.

28. Hirschfield RMA, Russell JM. Current concepts: assessment and treatment of suicidal patients [review]. N Engl J Med 1997;337:910–5.

29. Moscicki EK. Gender differences in completed and attempted suicides. Ann Epidemiol 1994;4:152–8.

30. Runeson BS. Mental disorder in youth suicide: DSM IIIR Axes I and II. Acta Psychiatr Scand 1989;79:490–7.

31. Mann JJ. A current perspective of suicide and attempted suicide. Ann Intern Med 2002;136:302–11.

32. Isometsa E, Henriksson M, Marttunen M, et al. Mental disorders in young and middle aged men who commit suicide. BMJ 1995;310:1366–7.

33. Jamison KR. Suicide and manic-depressive illness: an overview and personal account. In: Jacobs DG, editor. The Harvard Medical School guide to suicide assessment and intervention. San Francisco: Jossey-Bass; 1999. p. 251–69.

34. Roy A. Suicide and psychiatric patients. Psychiatr Clin North Am 1985;8:227–41.

35. Shaffer D, Garland A, Gould M, et al. Preventing teenage suicide: a critical review. J Am Acad Child Adolesc Psychiatry 1988;27:675–87.

36. Hawton K. Assessment of suicide risk. Br J Psychiatry 1987;150:145–53.

37. Brendel RW, Perlis R, Stern TA. Suicide. In: Stern TA, Rosenbaum JF, Fava M, et al, editors. Massachusetts General Hospital comprehensive clinical psychiatry. Philadelphia: Mosby/Elsevier; 2008. p. 733–45.

38. Abram HS, Moore GL, Westervelt FB. Suicidal behavior in chronic renal patients. Am J Psychiatry 1971;127:1199–204.

39. Kelly MJ, Mufson MJ, Rogers MP. Medical settings and suicide. In: Jacobs DG, editor. The Harvard Medical School guide to suicide assessment and intervention. San Francisco: Jossey-Bass; 1999. p. 491–519.

40. Marzuk PM, Tierney H, Tardiff K, et al. Increased risk of suicide in persons with AIDS. JAMA 1988;259:1333–7.
41. Hoffmann DP, Dubovsky SL. Depression and suicide assessment. Emerg Med Clin North Am 1991;9:107–21.
42. Roy A, Segal NL, Centerwall BS, et al. Suicide in twins. Arch Gen Psychiatry 1991;48:29–32.
43. Phillips DP, Cartensen LL. Clustering of teenage suicides after television news stories about suicide. N Engl J Med 1986;315:685–9.
44. Joiner TE Jr, Brown JS, Wingate LR. The psychology and neurobiology of suicidal behavior. Annu Rev Psychol 2005;56:287–314.
45. Smith JC, Mercy JA, Conn JM. Marital status and the risk of suicide. Am J Public Health 1988;78:78–80.
46. Buda M, Tsuang MT. The epidemiology of suicide: implications for clinical practice. In: Blumenthal SJ, Kupfer DJ, editors. Suicide over the life cycle: risk factors, assessment and treatment of suicidal patients. Washington, DC: American Psychiatric Press; 1990. p. 17–37.
47. Brent DA, Perper JA, Allman CJ, et al. The presence and accessibility of firearms in the homes of adolescent suicides: a case-controlled study. JAMA 1991;266:2989–95.
48. Buzan RD, Weissberg MP. Suicide: risk factors and therapeutic considerations in the emergency department. J Emerg Med 1992;10:33–43.
49. Heikkinen M, Aro H, Lonnqvist J. Recent life events, social support and suicide. Acta Psychiatr Scand 1994;377(Suppl):65–72.
50. Brent DA, Perper JA, Goldstein CE, et al. Risk factors for adolescent suicide. Arch Gen Psychiatry 1988;45:581–8.
51. Kellermann AL, Rivara FP, Somes G, et al. Suicide in the home in relationship to gun ownership. N Engl J Med 1992;327:467–72.
52. Goldstein RB, Black DW, Nasrallah A, et al. The prediction of suicide: sensitivity, specificity, and predictive value of a multivariate model applied to suicide among 1906 patients with affective disorders. Arch Gen Psychiatry 1991;48:418–22.
53. Hepp U, Moergeli H, Trier S, et al. Attempted suicide: factors leading to hospitalization. Can J Psychiatry 2004;49:736–42.
54. American Psychiatric Association. Practice guideline for the assessment and treatment of patients with suicidal behaviors. Am J Psychiatry 2003;160(11 Suppl):1–60.
55. Shuster JL, Lagomasino IT, Okereke OI, et al. Suicide. In: Irwin RS, Rippe JM, editors. Intensive care medicine. 5th edition. Philadelphia: Lippincott-Raven; 2003. p. 2184–9.
56. Blumenthal SJ. Suicide: a guide to risk factors, assessment, and treatment of suicidal patients. Med Clin North Am 1988;72:937–71.
57. Tsuang MT, Fleming JA, Simpson JC. Suicide and schizophrenia. In: Jacobs DG, editor. The Harvard Medical School guide to suicide assessment and intervention. San Francisco (CA): Jossey-Bass; 1999. p. 287–99.
58. Weisman AD, Worden JW. Risk-rescue rating in suicide assessment. Arch Gen Psychiatry 1972;26:553–60.
59. Miller MC. Suicide-prevention contracts: advantages, disadvantages and an alternative approach. In: Jacobs DG, editor. The Harvard Medical School guide to suicide assessment and intervention. San Francisco (CA): Jossey-Bass; 1999. p. 463–81.
60. Tondo L, Hennen J, Baldessarini RJ. Lower suicide risk with long-term lithium treatment in major affective illness: a meta-analysis. Acta Psychiatr Scand 2001;104:163–72.

61. Baldessarini RJ, Tondo L, Hennen J. Lithium treatment and suicide risk in major affective disorders: update and new findings. J Clin Psychiatry 2003;64(Suppl 5): 44–52.

62. Meltzer HY, Alphs L, Green AI, et al. Clozapine treatment for suicidality in schizophrenia: international suicide prevention trial (InterSePT). Arch Gen Psychiatry 2003;60:82–91.

63. Meltzer HY, Okayli G. Reduction of suicidality during clozapine treatment of neuroleptic-resistant schizophrenia: impact on risk-benefit assessment. Am J Psychiatry 1995;152:183–90.

64. Maltsberger JT. The psychodynamic understanding of suicide. In: Jacobs DG, editor. The Harvard Medical School guide to suicide assessment and intervention. San Francisco (CA): Jossey-Bass; 1999. p. 72–82.

65. Stern TA, Prager LM, Cremens MC. Autognosis rounds for medical housestaff. Psychosomatics 1993;34:1–7.

66. Leong GB, Silva JA, Weinstock R. Dangerousness. In: Rosner R, editor. Principles and practice of forensic psychiatry. 2nd edition. London: Arnold; 2003. p. 564–71.

67. Silver E, Mulvey EP, Monahan J. Assessing violence risk among discharged psychiatric patients: toward an ecological approach. Law Hum Behav 1999; 23:237–55.

68. Mossman D. Assessing predictions of violence: being accurate about accuracy. J Consult Clin Psychol 1994;62(4):783–92.

69. Steadman HJ. From dangerousness to risk assessment of community violence: taking stock at the turn of the century. J Am Acad Psychiatry Law 2000;28:265–71.

70. Beck JC, Schouten R. Workplace violence and psychiatric practice. Bull Menninger Clin 2000;64(1):36–48.

71. Gross AF, Sanders KM. Aggression and violence. In: Stern TA, Rosenbaum JF, Fava M, et al, editors. Massachusetts General Hospital comprehensive clinical psychiatry. Philadelphia: Mosby; 2008. p. 895–905.

72. Norko MA, Baranoski MV. The state of contemporary risk assessment research. Can J Psychiatry 2005;50:18–26.

73. Norko MA, Baranoski MV. The prediction of violence; detection of dangerousness. Brief Treat Crisis Interv 2008;8:73–91.

74. Elbogen EB, Johnson SC. The intricate link between violence and mental disorder: results from the national epidemiologic survey on alcohol and related conditions. Arch Gen Psychiatry 2009;66(2):152–61.

75. Swanson JW, Holzer CE, Gangu VK, et al. Violence and psychiatric disorder in the community: evidence from the Epidemiologic Catchment Area Surveys. Hosp Community Psychiatry 1990;41:761–70.

76. Monahan J, Steadman HJ, Robbins PC, et al. Developing a clinically useful actuarial tool for assessing violence risk. Br J Psychiatry 2000;176:312–9.

77. Friedman RA. Violence and mental illness – how strong is the link? N Engl J Med 2006;355(20):2064–6.

78. Swanson JW, Swartz MS, Essock SM, et al. The social-environmental context of violent behavior in persons treated for severe mental illness. Am J Public Health 2002;92(9):1523–31.

79. Steadman H, Mulvey E, Monahan J, et al. Violence by people discharged from acute psychiatric inpatient facilities and by others in the same neighborhoods. Arch Gen Psychiatry 1998;55(5):393–401.

80. Fulweiler C, Grossman H, Frobes C, et al. Early onset substance abuse and community violence by outpatients with chronic mental illness. Psychiatr Serv 1997;48:1181–5.

81. Johnson JG, Cohen P, Smailes E, et al. Adolescent personality disorders associated with violence and criminal behavior during adolescence and early adulthood. Am J Psychiatry 2000;157:1406–12.
82. Porter S, Woodworth M. Psychopathy and aggression. paperback edition 2007. In: Patrick CJ, editor. Handbook of psychopathy. New York: Guilford Press; 2006. p. 481–94.
83. Douglas KS, Vincent GM, Edens JF. Risk for criminal recidivism: the role of psychopathy. paperback edition 2007. In: Patrick CJ, editor. Handbook of psychopathy. New York: Guilford Press; 2006. p. 533–54.
84. Dolan M, Doyle M. Violence risk prediction. Br J Psychiatry 2000;177:303–11.
85. Tengstrom A, Grann M, Langstrom N, et al. Psychopathy (PCL-R) as a predictor of violent recidivism among criminal offenders with schizophrenia. Law Hum Behav 2000;24:45–58.
86. Link BG, Andrews H, Cullen FT. The violent and illegal behavior of mental patients reconsidered. Am Sociol Rev 1992;57:275–92.
87. Swanson JW, Borum R, Swartz M, et al. Psychotic symptoms and disorders and the risk of violent behavior in the community. Crim Behav Ment Health 1996;6: 317–38.
88. McNeil DE, Eisner JP, Binder RL. The relationship between command hallucinations and violence. Psychiatr Serv 2000;51:1288–92.
89. Link BG, Stueve A, Phelan J. Psychotic symptoms and violent behaviors: probing the components of threat/control/override symptoms. Soc Psychiatry Psychiatr Epidemiol 1998;33:S55–61.
90. Appelbaum PS, Robbins PC, Monahan J. Violence and delusions: data from the McArthur Violence Risk Assessment Study. Am J Psychiatry 2000;157: 566–72.
91. Steadman HJ, Silver E, Monahan J, et al. A classification tree approach to the development of actuarial violence risk assessment tools. Law Hum Behav 2000;24:83–100.
92. Walsh E, Buchanan A, Fahy T. Violence and schizophrenia: examining the evidence. Br J Psychiatry 2002;180:490–5.
93. Borum R, Swartz M, Swanson J. Assessing and managing violence risk in clinical practice. J Prac Psych Behav Health 1996;4:205–15.
94. Swanson JW, Swartz MS, VanDorn RA, et al. A national study of violent behavior in persons with schizophrenia. Arch Gen Psychiatry 2006;63:490–9.
95. Beck J, Baxter P. The violent patient. In: Lifson LE, Simon RI, editors. The mental health practitioner and the law. A comprehensive handbook. 1st edition. London: Harvard University Press; 1998.
96. Kaplan MS, Geling O. Firearm suicides and homicides in the United States: regional variations from patterns of gun ownership. Soc Sci Med 1998;46:1227–33.
97. Henry B, Moffitt TE. Neuropsychological and neuroimaging studies of juvenile delinquency and adult criminal behavior. In: Stoff D, Breiling J, Maser J, editors. Handbook of antisocial behavior. New York: John Wiley & Sons; 1997. p. 280–8.
98. Skeem JL, Schubert C, Odgers C, et al. Psychiatric symptoms and community violence among high-risk patients: a test of the relationship at the weekly level. J Consult Clin Psychol 2006;74:967–79.
99. Nestor PG. Mental disorder and violence: personality dimensions and clinical features. Am J Psychiatry 2002;159:1973–8.
100. Swartz MS, Swanson JW, Hiday VA, et al. Taking the wrong drugs; the role of substance abuse and medication non-compliance in violence among severely mentally ill individuals. Soc Psychiatry Psychiatr Epidemiol 1998;33(1):S75–80.

101. Elbogen EB, VanDorn RA, Swanson JW, et al. Treatment engagement and violence risk in mental disorders. Br J Psychiatry 2006;189:354–60.
102. Hare RD. The Hare Psychopathy Checklist – revised manual. Toronto: Multi Health Systems; 2003.
103. Harris GT, Rice ME, Quinsey VL. Violent recidivism of mentally disordered offenders: the development of a statistical prediction instrument. Crim Justice Behav 1993;20:315–35.
104. Dolan M, Doyle M. Clinical and actuarial measures and the role of the Psychopathy Checklist. Br J Psychiatry 2000;177:307–11.
105. Hart SD, Cox DN, Hare RD. The Hare Psychopathy Checklist: screening version (PCL-SV). Toronto: Multi-Health Systems; 1995.
106. Douglas KS, Ogloff JRP, Hart SD. Evaluation of a model of violence risk assessment among forensic psychiatric patients. Psychiatr Serv 2003;54:1372–9.
107. Mulvey EP, Lidz CW. Clinical prediction of violence as a conditional judgment. Soc Psychiatry Psychiatr Epidemiol 1998;33:S107–13.
108. Lidz CW, Mulvey EP, Gardner W. The accuracy of predictions of violence towards others. JAMA 1993;269:1007–111.
109. McNeil DE, Gregory AL, Lam JN, et al. Utility of decision support tools for assessing acute risk of violence. J Consult Clin Psychol 2003;71:945–53.
110. Dolan M, Doyle M. Violence risk prediction: clinical and actuarial measures and the role of the Psychopathy Checklist. Br J Psychiatry 2000;177:303–11.
111. Webster CD, Douglas KS, Eaves D, et al. HCR-20: Assessing risk for violence (version 2). Canada. Burnaby, BC: Mental Health Law, and Policy Institute, Simon Fraser University; 1997.
112. Monahan J, Steadman HJ, Robbins PC, et al. An actuarial model of violence risk assessment for persons with mental disorders. Psychiatr Serv 2005;56:810–5.
113. Dvoskin JA. Knowledge is not power, knowledge is obligation. J Am Acad Psychiatry Law 2002;30:533–40.

An Approach to the Patient with Cognitive Impairment: Delirium and Dementia

Jason P. Caplan, MD[a,b,]*, Terry Rabinowitz, MD, DDS[c,d]

KEYWORDS

- Cognitive impairment • Dementia
- Diagnostic criteria • Delirium

Reading the diagnostic criteria for the various psychiatric disorders that present with cognitive impairment may lead to the misperception that diagnosis is relatively easy to achieve when dealing with the cognitively impaired patient because this population can be divided into 2 broad groups: those with chronic cognitive decline (most likely diagnosable with a dementia) and those with acute cognitive changes (most likely experiencing a delirium). As is often the case, diagnosis in clinical practice is far more complicated than it is in textbooks.

Perhaps the greatest hurdle in evaluating the cognitively impaired patient is the clarification of a cohesive history. As the choice of one diagnosis over another may hinge almost entirely on the chronicity of symptoms, gaining some insight to this aspect of the patient's illness is vital. Unfortunately, the cognitively impaired patient is most often unable to provide such a history, and in the absence of a reliable family member, friend, or caregiver to fill in the gaps, diagnostic clarity can be difficult to achieve.

In this article, the authors outline the broad diagnostic spectra of delirium and dementia, review current understanding of their pathogenesis, and discuss useful diagnostic and therapeutic techniques.

DELIRIUM

Delirium is likely the most frequent cause of acute-onset cognitive impairment in the inpatient general hospital setting. Unfortunately, delirium is often either mis- or

[a] St Joseph's Hospital and Medical Center, 350 West Thomas Road, Phoenix, AZ 85013, USA
[b] Creighton University School of Medicine, Omaha, NE 68178, USA
[c] Division of Consultation Psychiatry and Psychosomatic Medicine and the Telemedicine, University of Vermont College of Medicine, Burlington, VT 05401, USA
[d] Fletcher Allen Health Care, 111 Colchester Avenue, Burlington, VT 05401, USA
* Corresponding author. Creighton University School of Medicine, Omaha, NE 68178.
E-mail address: jpcaplan@gmail.com

Med Clin N Am 94 (2010) 1103–1116
doi:10.1016/j.mcna.2010.08.004
0025-7125/10/$ – see front matter © 2010 Elsevier Inc. All rights reserved.

medical.theclinics.com

undiagnosed due to more prominent symptoms that obscure the detection of the cognitive decline. From a psychiatric perspective, delirium has been called "the great imitator" by virtue of clinicians frequently mistaking it for depression (due to patients appearing quiet or withdrawn), mania (due to agitation or sleep disturbance), psychosis (due to hallucinations or other perceptual disturbances), or anxiety (due to restlessness or fearfulness).[1] Indeed, studies of general hospital psychiatric consultation services have demonstrated misdiagnosis of delirium by nonpsychiatric hospital staff in at least 46% of cases.[2,3]

Delirium is a common complication of general hospital admission, presenting in 31% of all patients being admitted to the intensive care unit (ICU) and in 82% of those requiring intubation and mechanical ventilation.[4,5] Delirium has been shown to independently predict a 39% increase in ICU cost per patient and a 31% increase in the cost of hospital care alone.[6]

Financial matters aside, timely identification of delirium is of paramount importance for several reasons. Primarily, delirium represents a somatic (or "medical") disturbance presenting with a variety of possible cognitive and psychiatric symptoms. Delirium may present before other symptoms manifest, thus serving as an "early warning system," alerting treaters to the presence of systemic illness. Early recognition of delirium allows for early intervention, potentially forestalling progression to more disturbing psychiatric symptoms and resultant agitation or aggression. Aside from the immediate risks that agitation poses for both patient and hospital staff alike, unchecked delirium has also been associated with the later development of posttraumatic stress disorder (PTSD) due to the experience of horrifying delusions and hallucinations.[7,8]

Clinical Presentation

As defined by the *Diagnostic and Statistical Manual of Mental Disorders*, fourth edition—text revision (DSM-IV-TR), delirium is a syndrome presenting with a disturbance of consciousness with deficits of attention and changes in cognition or perception that develop over a short period and fluctuate over the course of the day.[9] The diagnosis also requires evidence from history, physical examination, or laboratory results that these findings are caused by an underlying medical condition. Of these features, inattention and the fluctuating (or waxing and waning) course are probably the most pathognomonic of the diagnosis. As already mentioned, the various "accessory" symptoms of delirium (eg, agitation, social withdrawal, fearfulness, flattening of affect, hallucinations, sleep disturbance) often result in misdiagnosis. No other psychiatric diagnosis presents with the inattention seen in delirium, leading many experts to identify this symptom as the hallmark of the condition. Indeed, bedside diagnosis often hinges on tests of attention.

Pathophysiology

Current understanding of the pathophysiology of delirium centers on a final common pathway of the effects of oxidative stress on the brain,[10] which allows for the hallmark features of delirium to present in cases with underlying somatic causes as diverse as urinary tract infection, traumatic brain injury, or drug reaction. Indeed, delirium may result from conditions spanning the entire breadth of medical practice. The immediately life-threatening causes of delirium can be remembered by the mnemonic "WHHHHIMPS" (**Box 1**).

It is theorized that because the neurons most vulnerable to oxidative stress are the dopaminergic and cholinergic ones, oxidative stress results in a state of hyperdopaminergia (due to release of endogenous dopamine) and hypocholinergia (due to loss

---

Box 1
WWHHHHHIMPS: A mnemonic for life-threatening causes of delirium

*W*ithdrawal

*W*ernicke encephalopathy

*H*ypoxia or hypoperfusion of the brain

*H*ypertensive crisis

*H*ypoglycemia

*H*yper- or hypothermia

*I*ntracranial hemorrhage or mass

*M*eningitis or encephalitis

*P*oisons (including medications)

*S*tatus epilepticus

Data from Wise MG, Trzepacz PT. Delirium (confusional states). In: Rundell JR, Wise MD, editors. The American psychiatric press textbook of consultation-liaison psychiatry. Washington, DC: American Psychiatric Press; 1996. p. 258–74.

---

of cholinergic transmission).[11] Excess dopamine results in hallucinations and agitation (because dopamine potentiates the action of the excitatory neurotransmitter glutamate), while a lack of acetylcholine leads to deficits of alertness and attention (because acetylcholine is the primary neurotransmitter of the reticular activating system that governs these functions via its projections to the thalami and inputs from the neocortex and limbic circuit).[12] Baseline deficits of cholinergic function in the elderly (particularly those already diagnosed with a dementia) are believed to underlie the increased risk of delirium in this population.

Diagnosis

Accurate diagnosis of delirium is typically made by bedside cognitive testing. The Mini-Mental State Examination (MMSE) has long been used as a brief and easily administered test of cognitive function, though some have criticized its use of serial 7s (counting back from 100 in intervals of 7) or spelling of "world" backward as tests of attention because they are too reliant on baseline level of education rather than current ability to attend.[13] Asking the patient to recite the days of the week and the months of the year in reverse order have been proposed as purer tests of attention, because almost every patient (regardless of educational achievement) can recite the days and months forward. The draw-a-clock task, in which the patient is presented with a circle drawn on a piece of paper and asked to fill in the numbers and to set the hands to a particular time (eg, ten to two), is also a method of bedside cognitive testing frequently used by general hospital psychiatrists to gauge multiple neuropsychiatric domains (including attention, planning, visuospatial reasoning, and impulsivity).[14]

In terms of diagnostic studies, perhaps no test is more reliable in the diagnosis of delirium than the electroencephalogram (EEG). Originally described by Engel and Romano more than 50 years ago, the classic EEG findings in delirium are generalized slowing to the theta-delta range, the consistency of this slowing regardless of underlying cause, and the resolution of this slowing with treatment.[15] The EEG may further delineate the underlying cause of the delirium if it reveals patterns characteristic of certain conditions (such as the rapid beta activity seen in sedative-hypnotic toxicity, triphasic waves associated with hepatic encephalopathy, or the periodic spike-wave discharges that occur with Creutzfeldt-Jakob disease).[16] The EEG is also, of course, the optimal diagnostic test to diagnose delirium that results from epilepsy (including partial complex status epilepticus and post-ictal conditions).

Because early recognition of delirium allows for more timely identification and treatment of the underlying cause, several scales have been developed and validated for use by nursing staff to enhance the detection of the condition. Perhaps the most commonly used is the Confusion Assessment Method (CAM), which also has a version refined for use in the ICU (CAM-ICU).[17,18] The abbreviated screening version of the CAM and the CAM-ICU focus on 4 cardinal symptoms of delirium, and can be administered rapidly at the bedside. The brevity of the tool allows for multiple assessments per day, an important quality given the inherent waxing and waning course of delirium (because diagnosis may be missed if the patient is "caught on the wane").

Treatment

The only definitive treatment for delirium is identification and resolution of the underlying cause. While such diagnostic and therapeutic efforts are under way there are approaches to the management of delirium that should be used. Given the hyperdopaminergic/hypocholinergic hypothesis of delirium, it makes sense that pharmacologic interventions should be directed to diminishing dopaminergic activity while optimizing cholinergic function.

Neuroleptics (originally developed for the treatment of schizophrenia) function primarily through the blockade of dopamine receptors and are thus a natural choice to accomplish the former of these goals. Of the neuroleptics, intravenous (IV) haloperidol has accumulated the greatest amount of data and empirical clinical experience supporting its efficacy and safety in the treatment of delirium, resulting from its regular use in this regard over the past 3 decades.[19] Haloperidol is a strong antagonist of the D_2 receptor and carries relatively little anticholinergic activity, thus limiting the hallucinations and agitation that result from endogenous dopamine release without exacerbating the deficits of alertness and attention due to hypocholinergia.[20] Indeed, it this combination of strong dopamine antagonism with negligible cholinergic activity (along with a low likelihood of inducing hypotension) that first prompted trials of IV haloperidol for management of the agitated delirious ICU patient.[1]

Although haloperidol has never received a formal Food and Drug Administration (FDA) indication for IV administration, it is considered the standard of care. An initial dose is typically in the range of 0.5 mg (for elderly patients) to 2 mg in cases of "quiet" delirium or mild agitation, though more significant agitation may require starting doses in the 5- to 10-mg range. Subsequent doses should occur after a 30-minute interval to allow for distribution of the medication (11 minutes in healthy subjects, typically longer in the medically ill).[21] If calm is not achieved with the initial dose, subsequent doses should be roughly doubled (ie, 1 mg, 2 mg, 5 mg, 10 mg, and so forth) until agitation is effectively managed. The effective dose can then be repeated on a 4- to 6-hour schedule with additional doses available as needed. Once calm has been maintained for a period of 24 hours, the regimen can be tapered.

As with most neuroleptic medications, chronic use of haloperidol has been associated with the development of extrapyramidal symptoms (EPS), however, these seem to be rare when the medication is administered IV.[22] Clinicians may also be loath to use haloperidol because of concerns of prolongation of the corrected QT interval (QTc) and the risk of torsades de pointes. It should be noted that of the commonly used neuroleptic medications, haloperidol is associated with among the lowest per-dose-equivalent prolongation of the QTc.[23] Furthermore, a large number of non-neuroleptic medications are also strongly associated with prolonged QTc, including antibiotics (fluororquinolones), antiarrhythmics (amiodarone, flecainide), and pain medications (methadone).[24] Nonetheless, care should be taken with the administration of IV haloperidol including close monitoring of the QTc (via telemetry if needed), regular assessment and requisite replenishment of potassium and magnesium (because hypokalemia and hypomagnesemia independently predispose to QTc prolongation), and potential replacement of other QTc prolonging agents if necessary.[1]

The development of parenteral formulations of the newer, so-called atypical neuroleptics has resulted in interest in their utility in the management of delirium. Of this group, risperidone has accumulated the most data indicating safety and efficacy in the treatment of delirium.[25] Some of the other drugs in this class (olanzapine, quetiapine, aripiprazole, and ziprasidone) have more limited supporting data, but some smaller studies have shown some potential benefit of their use. All of these drugs, however, are limited to oral or intramuscular (IM) (for olanzapine and ziprasidone) administration. When faced with a confused and potentially agitated patient, oral dosing may not be an option, and repeated painful IM injections are unlikely to create the desired sense of calm or therapeutic trust. Quetiapine and clozapine occupy a niche role in the treatment of patients with Parkinson disease or dementia with Lewy bodies who become delirious, because the minimal antagonism of these drugs at the dopamine receptor is less likely to exacerbate their underlying parkinsonian symptoms.[26]

Although there are several agents available to address the first half of the hyperdopaminergic/hypocholinergic hypothesis, there is very little evidence that medications intended to increase cholinergic transmission are useful in the management of delirium. Small studies of the cholinesterase inhibitors approved for the treatment of dementia have shown some potential delirioprotective effect,[27] but randomized, double-blind, placebo-controlled trials have failed to demonstrate any benefit of these agents in either preventing or treating postoperative delirium.[28,29] Physostigmine has proved efficacious in reversing delirium from several causes, but due to a narrow therapeutic window and brief duration of effect, its use is limited to presentations of delirium due to anticholinergic poisoning.[30]

Prevention

Because delirium is a systemic manifestation of a somatic illness, definitive prevention of delirium would require prevention of all illness and injury. More realistically, we can limit agents and interventions that place our patients at greater risk for delirium, because in most cases, delirium results from a series of stressors placed on the body and brain rather that a single "hit." Perhaps most easily managed are the medications administered to patients that may result in delirium. While almost all medications can provoke delirium, the "usual suspects" often include anticholinergics, opiates, and benzodiazepines. Limiting the doses of the medications or replacing them with less deliriogenic alternatives can be of great benefit to the patient.

To that end, recent studies have demonstrated that dexmedetomidine (a centrally acting α_2-adrenergic agonist sedative-analgesic agent) is significantly less likely to result in delirium than either midazolam or propofol when used as a postoperative sedative for mechanical ventilation.[31,32] In addition, a recent large (N = 400) randomized, double-blind, placebo-controlled study of olanzapine and placebo in elderly patients with joint replacement revealed that 10 mg of olanzapine administered perioperatively reduced the incidence of postoperative delirium (from 40% to 14%) and increased the likelihood of discharge to home (vs a rehabilitation facility).[33] Other strategies to prevent or minimize the consequences of delirium are under way.

DEMENTIA

According to DSM-IV-TR, the essential feature of a dementia is the development of multiple cognitive deficits that *must* include memory impairment and at least one other cognitive disturbance including aphasia, apraxia, agnosia, or a disturbance of executive function. In addition (and of particular importance to this article), the diagnosis of dementia should not be made if the cognitive deficits occur *exclusively* during the course of a delirium. Although this is a potentially helpful way to differentiate between delirium and dementia, it is not uncommon for a patient with dementia to present with an acute onset of confusion (ie, delirium) because dementia is an independent risk factor for development of delirium. Therefore, this combination of conditions may be especially perplexing with respect to presentation, etiology, and treatment. From a practical perspective, however, the key features that may help to differentiate between delirium and dementia include the following: the cognitive deficits in dementia are generally chronic and develop slowly; the onset of cognitive deficits in delirium are much more acute; a "pure" dementia early in its course occurs in the presence of a clear sensorium; and a reduced ability to sustain or shift attention makes the diagnosis of delirium more likely. When evaluating a patient for dementia, it may be useful to view the condition as more than a cognitive disorder. In addition to cognitive deficits, disturbances in daily function and behavior as well as neurologic changes should be evaluated and tracked over time to serve as aids to diagnosis and response to treatment.[34]

Types of Dementia

Dementia of the Alzheimer type or Alzheimer disease (AD) is the most common type of dementia, with a prevalence in those at age 65 years of approximately 1 per 100 individuals. This prevalence doubles with every 5-year increment or increase in age. Diagnostic criteria for AD include the "core" symptoms of dementia, namely a major impairment of learning, retaining, or recalling information and at least one of the following: aphasia, apraxia, agnosia, or disturbance in executive function (ie, planning, organizing, sequencing, or abstracting). The cognitive deficits must cause significant impairment in social or occupational function and represent a significant decline from a previous level of function. The course of the disorder is characterized by a gradual onset and by continuing cognitive decline. The average duration from onset of symptoms to death is 8 to 10 years. Disorders that must be ruled out before AD can be diagnosed include cerebrovascular disease, Parkinson disease, Huntington disease, normal-pressure hydrocephalus, hypothyroidism, B_{12} or folic acid deficiency, neurosyphilis, human immunodeficiency virus infection, and substance-induced cognitive impairment.

The 2 most important risk factors for development of AD include advancing age (after age 85 years the risk is as high as 50%) and a first-degree biologic relative with the early-onset type of AD (ie, with an onset before the age of 65 years). Additional risk factors include presence of the apolipoprotein-e4 (APOE-e4) gene, a history of head injury (even remote history), cardiovascular disease (including atherosclerosis, stroke, hypertension, or carotid artery disease), elevated levels of homocysteine, and very low educational achievement (ie, < an eighth-grade education). Protective factors include use of nonsteroidal anti-inflammatory drugs (NSAIDs), wine consumption (in moderation), coffee consumption, and regular physical activity.[35,36] These factors should be carefully considered because some studies have found no increased risk for AD in those with a family history of dementia, or a history of depression, estrogen replacement therapy, head trauma, smoking, hypertension, heart disease, or stroke.[35] Psychiatric or behavioral disturbances in AD are common and include depression, anxiety, agitation (including physical aggressiveness and wandering), sleep disturbances, delusions, and hallucinations.

A diagnosis of AD may be confirmed at autopsy. Its characteristic microscopic findings include neuritic plaques (NPs; also called senile plaques) and neurofibrillary tangles (NFTs). The NPs are generated by a deposition of fibrils of the β-amyloid peptide, Aβ, a fragment derived from the proteolysis of amyloid precursor protein (APP), in the brain. NFTs are composed of paired helical filaments (PHFs), which are composed of the microtubule-associated protein tau. In NFTs, tau is excessively phosphorylated, which leads to the aggregation of tau molecules and their ultimate transition to insoluble NFTs.[36,37] AD is the quintessential cortical dementia (**Table 1**). A helpful mnemonic to remember the characteristics of a cortical dementia is the "4 As": amnesia, apraxia, aphasia, and agnosia; in comparison, subcortical dementia is characterized by defects in arousal, attention, motivation, and the rate of information processing.[38]

Vascular dementia (also called multi-infarct dementia or vascular cognitive disorder) is characterized by cognitive deficits thought to be etiologically related to cerebrovascular disease, as demonstrated by either focal neurologic signs and symptoms or laboratory findings. Although overall it is the second most common type of dementia, comprising 10% to 20% of all dementia cases, it is much less common than AD.[39] In most cases the onset of symptoms is abrupt, but some patients may have so-called silent strokes that at first do not present with obvious signs and symptoms. As more areas of the brain become damaged, symptoms begin to appear. The disease is more common in men than women.[40]

Table 1
Comparison of delirium and dementia

Feature	Delirium	Dementia
Onset	Abrupt	Usually insidious; abrupt in some strokes/trauma
Course	Fluctuates	Slow decline
Duration	Hours to weeks	Months to years
Attention	Impaired	Intact early; often impaired late
Sleep-wake	Disrupted	Usually normal
Alertness	Impaired	Normal
Orientation	Impaired	Intact early; impaired late
Behavior	Agitated, withdrawn/depressed, or both	Intact early
Speech	Incoherent, rapid/slowed	Word-finding problems
Thoughts	Disorganized, delusions	Impoverished
Perceptions	Hallucinations/illusions	Usually intact early

Data from Butler C, Zeman AZJ. Neurologic syndromes which can be mistaken for psychiatric conditions. J Neurol Neurosurg Psychiatry 2005;76:i31–8; Rabinowitz T. Delirium: an important (but often unrecognized) clinical syndrome. Curr Psychiatry Rep 2002;4:202–8; and Rabinowitz T, Murphy KM, Nagle KJ, et al. Delirium: pathophysiology, recognition, prevention and treatment. Expert Rev Neurotherapeutics 2003;3:89–101.

Diagnostic criteria for vascular dementia include the core criteria for dementia listed above. In addition, focal neurologic signs and symptoms or laboratory evidence of cerebrovascular disease felt to be etiologically related to the disorder must be present. These indicators include exaggeration of deep tendon reflexes, gait abnormalities, weakness of an extremity, and imaging studies that demonstrate multiple infarctions of the cortex and underlying white matter.

Risk factors for vascular dementia include male gender; African American ethnicity; hypertension; history of stroke, diabetes, and heart disease; and high cholesterol levels. Psychiatric or behavioral symptoms include depression, apathy, mania, anxiety, emotional lability, agitation, psychosis, and delusions. Vascular dementia is the most common type of mixed dementia; it presents with signs and symptoms of both cortical and subcortical dementia (**Table 2**).

Dementia with Lewy bodies (DLB) is the second most common type of dementia in the elderly. DLB is characterized by marked impairments in visuospatial, attentional, and executive functions, and may be differentiated from AD because DLB often presents with relatively well-preserved memory in its early stages. Additional features of DLB include persistent, well-formed visual hallucinations in up to 80% of cases, and parkinsonism.[41] Lewy bodies are intranuclear collections of α-synuclein protein in the neurons in brain regions responsible for memory and motor control. Furthermore,

Table 2
Characteristics of cortical and subcortical dementia

Characteristic or Function	Cortical eg, Dementia in Alzheimer Disease or Pick Disease	Subcortical eg, Dementia in Huntington Disease, Parkinson Disease, or HIV Infection
Alertness	Normal	"Slowed up"
Attention	Normal early	Impaired
Language	Aphasia early	No aphasia
Episodic memory	Amnesia	Forgetfulness
Visuospatial skills	Impaired	Impaired
Calculation	Involved early	Preserved until late
Personality	Unconcerned or disinhibited if frontal type, otherwise preserved	Apathetic, inert
Mood	Euthymic	Depressed
Speech	Normal articulation	Dysarthric
Movement disorders	Absent	Common
Pathology	Primary damage to neocortex and hippocampus	Primary damage to deep gray matter and white matter structures, including the thalamus, basal ganglia, brainstem nuclei, and frontal lobe projections

Data from Gray KF, Cummings JL. Dementia. In: Wise MG, Rundell JR, editors. The American psychiatric publishing textbook of consultation-liaison psychiatry. Washington, DC: American Psychiatric Publishing Inc; 2002. p. 273–306; Butler C, Zeman AZJ. Neurologic syndromes which can be mistaken for psychiatric conditions. J Neurol Neurosurg Psychiatry 2005;76:i31–8; and Lavretsky H, Chui HC. Vascular dementia. In: Agronin ME, Maletta GJ, editors. Principles and practice of geriatric psychiatry. Philadelphia: Lippincott Williams & Wilkins; 2006. p. 301–10.

DLB may produce a waxing and waning pattern of cognitive impairment similar to that seen in delirium, thus rendering accurate diagnosis more difficult.

Dementia associated with depression or other psychiatric disorders is often incorrectly referred to as pseudodementia. However, the cognitive deficits caused by an underlying psychiatric condition may be indistinguishable from those in primary dementia and are quite real; the major difference between the 2 conditions is that dementia associated with a psychiatric condition improves or completely resolves with successful treatment (usually with an antidepressant medication, although some severe cases may require electroconvulsive therapy).

Dementia occurs in up to 40% of patients with *Parkinson disease* (PD), a condition characterized by progressive neurodegenerative disease that includes cardinal motor symptoms of bradykinesia, resting tremor, rigidity, and impaired postural reflexes due to loss of pigmented dopaminergic neurons in the substantia nigra pars compacta (SNpc).[42,43] In some cases, cognitive and intellectual decline will not meet the full criteria for dementia; the most commonly affected domain, that of executive function, manifests as forgetfulness, poor attention, absent-mindedness, or disorganization. The mean time from onset of PD to dementia is approximately 10 years.[44]

Reversible dementias are dementias that may resolve after appropriate therapy. There are many potential causes, and it is recommended that (even in situations where it is highly likely that a dementia is due to an "irreversible" cause, such as AD) other treatable causes be sought as it is possible that presenting symptoms may result from overlapping conditions. Causes of reversible dementias include, but are not limited to, vitamin (eg, B_1, B_{12}, folate, niacin) deficiencies, endocrine (eg, adrenal, parathyroid, thyroid) dysfunction, anemia, medications (eg, anticholinergic agents, H_2 blockers, psychotropics), and paraneoplastic phenomena.

Dementia may be a component of many other conditions or insults including Huntington disease, Wilson disease, Pick disease, Creutzfeldt-Jakob disease, progressive supranuclear palsy, chronic substance abuse, and head trauma. Because both dementia and delirium are due to one or more medical conditions, clinicians should perform a thorough "rule-out" of likely (and sometimes not so likely) causes of these conditions to make certain that reversible or treatable causes are not overlooked. **Table 1** summarizes the clinical features useful in the differentiation of delirium and dementia.

Treatment or Management

The strategies for treatment or management of dementia may be divided into 2 broad categories: pharmacologic and nonpharmacologic (ie, behavioral). As is true for delirium, a methodical step-wise approach is the best tactic, aimed at identifying all potentially reversible or treatable causes and addressing each one. An example of this first step might be suspecting that a dementia is due to a hypothyroid state: the approach here would be to normalize thyroid function and observe for improvement. In practical terms, this is unlikely to be of much immediate help given that it may take days to weeks for thyroid function to improve and other interventions not specifically aimed at the suspected cause of the dementia will be necessary.

To date, few medications can effectively target specific chemical "deficiencies" or "surpluses" in the central nervous system with dementia (**Table 3**). However, because there is convincing evidence that both the cholinergic and glutamatergic systems are dysregulated in AD, important exceptions are 2 drug classes (acetylcholinesterase inhibitors [AChEIs] and glutamate modulators) that are effective in AD.[45] In addition, there is growing evidence that both classes may be beneficial in vascular dementia[46–48] and in DLB.[49,50] Currently available AChEIs include donepezil,

Table 3
Some recommended drug classes for treatment of co-occurring symptoms in dementia

Symptom	Drug Class	Comments
Agitation	Atypical antipsychotic; benzodiazepine; trazodone	Atypical antipsychotics are less likely to cause EPS; any antipsychotic may cause severe/fatal reactions in DLB (clozapine and quetiapine have lowest risk due to low affinity for the dopamine receptor); not approved for dementia-related psychosis—increased mortality risk; trazodone may cause orthostasis/"hangover"
Anxiety	Antidepressants (SNRI; SSRI; TCA); benzodiazepines	Benzodiazepines may cause disinhibition in some patients
Cognitive dysfunction	AChEI, memantine	
Depression	SNRI; SSRI; TCA	TCAs are less desirable due to their anticholinergic potential
Mania or disinhibition	CBZ, VPA	May cause nausea or excessive sedation
Psychosis	Atypical antipsychotics	Atypical antipsychotics are less likely to cause EPS; any antipsychotic may cause severe/fatal reactions in DLB; not approved for dementia-related psychosis—increased mortality risk
Sleep disturbance	Trazodone, benzodiazepines, eszopiclone, zaleplon, zolpidem	Eszopiclone, zaleplon, and zolpidem carry a risk of worsening confusion, hallucinations, and sleep behavior disorders

Abbreviations: AChEI, acetylcholinesterase inhibitor; CBZ, carbamazepine; DLB, dementia with Lewy bodies; EPS, extrapyramidal symptoms; SNRI, serotonin-norepinephrine reuptake inhibitor; SSRI, selective serotonin reuptake inhibitor; TCA, tricyclic antidepressant; VPA, valproic acid.

galantamine, and rivastigmine; all have beneficial effects on mild to moderate AD, although many clinicians (sometimes due to pressure from family members) prescribe these medications for severe disease or continue them in the presence of worsening symptoms. However, benefit is limited to slowing down the progression of the disease; it does not cure the condition. Likewise, memantine, the only available glutamate modulator, is effective in moderate to severe AD by delaying disease progression.[51] It is not uncommon for both an AChEI and memantine to be prescribed at the same time.[52,53]

Pharmacotherapy for the other dementias, as well as for the behavioral changes accompanying AD, DLB, and vascular dementia, is generally aimed at co-occurring signs and symptoms (such as agitation, anxiety, depression, hallucinations, and delusions); it typically involves the use of drug classes commonly identified for these conditions (see **Table 3**).

Behavioral interventions for dementia may be as or more important than pharmacologic approaches. This therapy should focus on keeping the affected patient as comfortable, safe, and free of physical restraint as possible and on maximizing the patient's dignity. Many of these interventions rely on family or other loved ones as well as on common sense for efficacy, and they include simple strategies (such as keeping the room well lit; using "orienting" items, such as a calendar or clock; placing pictures of well-known family members/friends/pets in the room; playing calming or well-known music; limiting the number of visitors to a few at a time to avoid "sensory overload"; making sure the affected patient has his or her eyeglasses and hearing aids on [and check the batteries in the hearing aids!]; keeping directions/explanations simple; straightforward, and unambiguous; avoiding excessive talk with other visitors that may lead to "defocusing" on the patient; visiting at times when the patient is at his or her best [eg, most alert, best pain control]; and allowing the patient plenty of rests and breaks from visitors).

SUMMARY

While identification of the cause of confusion in the cognitively impaired patient is important to guide further workup and prognosis, the care of this group of patients has a strong central theme. Whether the patient is suffering from a delirium or a dementia, their care calls for a careful step-wise approach to identifying and addressing somatic issues that may be either directly causing (in the case of delirium) or exacerbating (in the case of dementia) cognitive and behavioral issues. Furthermore, the environmental and behavioral cues discussed here can be of great benefit to many of these patients. Clinicians will do well by following these recommendations and additionally by helping to support the affected patient's caregiver(s) through education, empowerment, and empathy.

REFERENCES

1. Caplan JP, Cassem NH, Murray GB, et al. Delirium. In: Stern TA, Rosenbaum JF, Fava M, et al, editors. Massachusetts General Hospital comprehensive clinical psychiatry. Philadelphia: Mosby; 2008. p. 217–29.
2. Armstrong SC, Cozza KL, Watanabe KS. The misdiagnosis of delirium. Psychosomatics 1997;38(5):433–9.
3. Swigart SE, Kishi Y, Thurber S, et al. Misdiagnosed delirium in patient referrals to a university-based hospital psychiatry department. Psychosomatics 2008;49(2): 104–8.
4. McNicoll L, Pisani MA, Zhang Y, et al. Delirium in the intensive care unit: occurrence and clinical course in older patients. J Am Geriatr Soc 2003;51:591–8.
5. Ely EW, Shintani A, Truman B, et al. Delirium as a predictor of mortality in mechanically ventilated patients in the intensive care unit. J Am Med Assoc 2004;291: 1753–62.
6. Milbrandt EB, Deppen S, Harrison PL, et al. Costs associated with delirium in mechanically ventilated patients. Crit Care Med 2004;32:955–62.
7. DiMartini A, Dew MA, Kormos R, et al. Posttraumatic stress disorder caused by hallucinations and delusions experienced in delirium. Psychosomatics 2007; 48(5):436–9.
8. Davydow DS, Gifford JM, Desai SV, et al. Posttraumatic stress disorder in general intensive care unit survivors: a systematic review. Gen Hosp Psychiatry 2008; 30(5):421–34.

9. American Psychiatric Association. Diagnostic and statistical manual of mental disorders, (DSM-IV). 4th edition. Washington, DC: American Psychiatric Association; 1994.

10. Seaman JS, Schillerstrom J, Carroll D, et al. Impaired oxidative metabolism precipitates delirium: a study of 101 ICU patients. Psychosomatics 2006;47: 56–61.

11. Brown TM. Basic mechanisms in the pathogenesis of delirium. In: Stoudemire A, Fogel BS, Greenberg D, editors. Psychiatric care of the medical patient. 2nd edition. New York: Oxford University Press; 2000. p. 571–80.

12. Querques J. An approach to acute changes in mental status. In: Stern TA, editor. The ten-minute guide to psychiatric diagnosis and treatment. New York: Professional Publishing Group; 2005. p. 97–107.

13. Folstein MF, Folstein SE, McHugh PR. Mini-Mental State, a practical method for grading the cognitive state of patients for the clinician. J Psychiatr Res 1975; 12:189–98.

14. Freedman M, Leach L, Kaplan E, et al. Clock drawing: a neuropsychological analysis. New York: Oxford University Press; 1994.

15. Engel G, Romano J. Delirium, a syndrome of cerebral insufficiency. J Chronic Dis 1959;9:260–77.

16. Jacobson S, Jerrier H. EEG in delirium. Semin Clin Neuropsychiatry 2000;5(2): 86–92.

17. Inouye SK, Van Dyke CH, Alessi CA, et al. Clarifying confusion: the Confusion assessment method. Ann Intern Med 1990;113:941–8.

18. Ely EW, Margolin R, Francis J, et al. Evaluation of delirium in critically ill patients: validation of the confusion assessment method for the intensive care unit (CAM-ICU). Crit Care Med 2001;29:1370–9.

19. Caplan JP. Haloperidol and delirium: management or treatment? Crit Care Med 2009;37(1):354–5.

20. Attard A, Ranjith G, Taylor D. Delirium and its treatment. CNS Drugs 2008;22(8): 631–44.

21. Forsman A, Ohman R. Pharmacokinetic studies on haloperidol in man. Curr Ther Res Clin Exp 1976;10:319.

22. Menza MA, Murray GB, Holmes VF, et al. Decreased extrapyramidal symptoms with intravenous haloperidol. J Clin Psychiatry 1987;48:278–80.

23. Glassman AH, Bigger JT Jr. Antipsychotic drugs: prolonged QTc interval, torsade de pointes, and sudden death. Am J Psychiatry 2001;158:1774–82.

24. Stöllberger C, Huber JO, Finsterer J. Antipsychotic drugs and QT prolongation. Int Clin Psychopharmacol 2005;20:243–51.

25. Peritogiannis V, Stefanou E, Lixouriotis C, et al. Atypical antipsychotics in the treatment of delirium. Psychiatry Clin Neurosci 2009;63(5):623–31.

26. Lauterbach EC. The neuropsychiatry of Parkinson's disease and related disorders. Psychiatr Clin North Am 2004;27:801–25.

27. Dautzenberg PL, Mulder LJ, Olde Rikkert MG, et al. Delirium in elderly hospitalized patients: protective effects of chronic rivastigmine usage. Int J Geriatr Psychiatry 2004;19(7):641–4.

28. Overshott R, Karim S, Burns A. Cholinesterase inhibitors for delirium. Cochrane Database Syst Rev 2008;1:CD005317.

29. Gamberini M, Bolliger D, Lurati Buse GA, et al. Rivastigmine for the prevention of postoperative delirium in elderly patients undergoing elective cardiac surgery—a randomized controlled trial. Crit Care Med 2009;37(5): 1762–8.

30. Burns MJ, Linden CH, Graudins A, et al. A comparison of physostigmine and benzodiazepines for the treatment of anticholinergic poisoning. Ann Emerg Med 2000;35:374–81.

31. Riker RR, Shehabi Y, Bokesch PM, et al. Dexmedetomidine vs midazolam for sedation of critically ill patients: a randomized trial. JAMA 2009;301(5): 489–99.

32. Maldonado JR, Wysong A, van der Starre PJ, et al. Dexmedetomidine and the reduction of postoperative delirium after cardiac surgery. Psychosomatics 2009;50(3):206–17.

33. Larsen KA, Kelly SE, Stern TA, et al. Administration of olanzapine to prevent post-operative delirium in elderly joint replacement patients: a randomized controlled trial. Psychosomatics 2010;51(5):409–18.

34. Boyle LL, Ismail MS, Porteinsson AP. The dementia workup. In: Agronin ME, Maletta GJ, editors. Principles and practice of geriatric psychiatry. Philadelphia: Lippincott Williams & Wilkins; 2006. p. 135–52.

35. Lindsay J, Laurin D, Verreault R, et al. Risk factors for Alzheimer's disease: a prospective analysis from the Canadian study of Health and Aging. Am J Epidemiol 2002;156:445–53.

36. Knopman D. Alzheimer's disease. In: Agronin ME, Maletta GJ, editors. Principles and practice of geriatric psychiatry. Philadelphia: Lippincott Williams and Wilkins; 2006. p. 283–300.

37. Maccioni RB, Munoz JP, Barbeito L. The molecular bases of Alzheimer's disease and other neurodegenerative disorders. Arch Med Res 2001;32:367–81.

38. Gray KF, Cummings JL. Dementia. In: Wise MG, Rundell JR, editors. The American psychiatric publishing textbook of consultation-liaison psychiatry. Washington, DC: American Psychiatric Publishing, Inc; 2002. p. 273–306.

39. Jellinger KA. The pathology of "vascular dementia": a critical update. J Alzheimers Dis 2008;14:107–23.

40. Health NIo: NINDS Multi-Infarct Dementia Information Page, 2010. Available at: http://www.ninds.nih.gov/disorders/multi_infarct_dementia/multi_infarct_dementia.htm. Accessed August 10, 2010.

41. Weisman D, McKeith I. Dementia with Lewy bodies. Semin Neurol 2007;27:42–7.

42. Hindle JV. Ageing, neurodegeneration and Parkinson's disease. Age ageing 2010;39:156–61.

43. Gabelle A, Portet F, Berr C, et al. Neurodegenerative dementia and parkinsonism. J Nutr Health Aging 2010;14:37–44.

44. Aarsland D, Kurz MW. The epidemiology of dementia associated with Parkinson's disease. J Neurol Sci 2010;289:18–22.

45. Lleo A, Greenberg SM, Growdon JH. Current pharmacotherapy for Alzheimer's disease. Annu Rev Med 2006;57:513–33.

46. Wong CL, Bansback N, Lee PE, et al. Cost-effectiveness: cholinesterase inhibitor and memantine in vascular dementia. Can J Neurol Sci 2009;36:735–9.

47. Farlow MR. Use of antidementia agents in vascular dementia: beyond Alzheimer disease. Mayo Clin Proc 2006;81:1350–8.

48. Burns A, O'Brien J, group BAPDC, et al. Clinical practice with anti-dementia drugs: a consensus statement from British Association for Psychopharmacology. J Psychopharmacol 2006;20:732–55.

49. Levin OS, Batukaeva LA, Smolentseva IG, et al. Efficacy and safety of memantine in Lewy body dementia. Neurosci Behav Physiol 2009;39:597–604.

50. Dodel R, Csoti I, Ebersbach G, et al. Lewy body dementia and Parkinson's disease with dementia. J Neurol 2008;225(Suppl 5):39–47.

51. Thomas SJ, Grossberg GT. Memantine: a review of studies into its safety and efficacy in treating Alzheimer's disease and other dementias. Clin Interv Aging 2009; 4:367–77.

52. Froelich L, Andreasen N, Tsolaki M, et al. Long-term treatment of patients with Alzheimer's disease in primary and secondary care: results from an international survey. Curr Med Res Opin 2009;25:3059–68.

53. Geerts H, Grossberg GT. Pharmacology of acetylcholinesterase inhibitors and N-methyl-D-aspartate receptors for combination therapy in the treatment of Alzheimer's disease. J Clin Pharmacol 2006;46:8S–16S.

An Approach to the Patient with Dysregulated Mood: Major Depression and Bipolar Disorder

John Querques, MD[a,b,]*, Nicholas Kontos, MD[a,b]

KEYWORDS

- Bipolar disorder • Major depressive disorder
- Dysregulated mood • Dysphoria

Major depressive disorder (MDD) and bipolar disorder are chronic, relapsing-remitting illnesses whose effects on mood, behavior, and thinking exact a heavy toll on patients' physical and mental health and on their capacity for satisfying relationships and employment. Recent estimates from a large epidemiologic survey of the 12-month prevalence of MDD and bipolar I and II disorders were 6.7% and 2.6%, respectively.[1] Although these numbers may not seem large, the bulk of these patients' treatment is rendered by primary care practitioners. The same study showed that psychiatrists provided 12.3% of these patients' care, nonpsychiatrist mental health professionals 16%, and general medical providers nearly 23%, almost twice that of the psychiatrists' proportion.[2] In the inpatient setting, these affective illnesses and their treatments can complicate the diagnosis, course, therapy, and prognosis of numerous medical conditions. In this article, the authors discuss a general approach for general internists, family practitioners, and other primary care providers to follow in caring for patients with suspected MDD or bipolar disorder. Treatment of these conditions is discussed in the article by Huffman and Alpert elsewhere in this issue.

APPROACH TO THE PATIENT WITH SUSPECTED MDD
Assessment of Dysphoria

The initial step in the differential diagnosis of patients who are thought to have MDD is to determine if the patients and their moods are best described as dysphoric. Early in

[a] Department of Psychiatry, Massachusetts General Hospital, 55 Fruit Street, Boston, MA 02114, USA
[b] Department of Psychiatry, Harvard Medical School, Boston, MA, USA
* Corresponding author. Department of Psychiatry, Massachusetts General Hospital, 55 Fruit Street, Boston, MA 02114.
E-mail address: jquerques@partners.org

Med Clin N Am 94 (2010) 1117–1126
doi:10.1016/j.mcna.2010.08.011
0025-7125/10/$ – see front matter © 2010 Elsevier Inc. All rights reserved.

medical.theclinics.com

the evaluation, it is useful to use the terms dysphoric, low, or dejected to describe the patient's mood state rather than depressed, which can imply that the diagnosis of MDD or another depressive disorder has already been made. Many patients, at first glance, look dysphoric and the diagnosis of MDD is often made before ensuring that dysphoria is actually the most accurate categorization of the patient's state. Such premature closure frequently occurs in patients with hypoactive delirium, dementia, apathy, demoralization, or oppression.

By virtue of psychomotor retardation and cognitive slowing, patients with dementia or hypoactive delirium can appear dysphoric. However, affective constriction is not the predominant problem in these patients and to stop there and miss the fundamental cognitive derangement in demented or delirious patients would lead to a misdiagnosis of MDD.

The patient with apathy suffers from a diminution not only in interests and emotions but also in motivation.[3] Initiative, goal-directed behavior, and emotional responsiveness are diminished. Asked if they are sad, these patients typically say, quite dispassionately, that they are not. It may be more accurate to say that an apathetic patient's mood is absent or blank rather than low or down. Apathy can be seen in Parkinson disease, frontal lobe injuries, and infarctions of the cingulate gyrus or right frontoparietal lobe.[3]

Overwhelmed by protracted illness or difficult treatment, the demoralized patient "is no longer able to bear up under adversity."[4] The adjectives disheartened, discouraged, and dejected are apt for describing such a patient. As opposed to MDD and similar to grief, demoralization is a normal understandable response.

Oppression may be a milder form of demoralization. Frustrated and angry, the oppressed patient is sick and tired of being sick and tired. The oppressed patient may make comments about dying (eg, "If I need to wait another day for that test, I'm gonna throw myself out the window"), which raise the specter of suicidal intent when, in fact, they are simply declarations of frustration. One way to visualize this scenario is to picture a person weighed down by a load on the shoulders. If the impression is that the patient can "bounce back" if the burden is removed, he or she is likely oppressed; if the impression is that the individual would still be hobbled even without the weight on the shoulders, he or she is likely depressed. Although the diagnosis of either of these conditions should not rely solely on this imagery, such mental visualization can nevertheless be quite helpful.

Assessment of Abnormality

Another critical factor to bear in mind is that even when a patient's mood is appropriately considered dysphoric, such an affective state can be normal, that is, part of everyday human experience. There can be a danger in pathologizing such normal experiences. For example, patients who are grieving the loss of a loved one are usually not happy. Both common sense and the text revision of the fourth edition of the *Diagnostic and Statistical Manual of Mental Disorders* (DSM-IV-TR)[5] exclude such patients from the diagnosis of MDD. Some investigators have argued that contemporary psychiatry is guilty of pathologizing "normal intense sadness" and that perhaps the so-called bereavement exclusion should be applied to other stressful conditions.[6,7] Such distinctions aim to respect the normal frailty and resilience of the human person in the face of adversity.

Low mood may be thought to be abnormal because it is severe or disproportionately enduring to its cause, associated with other symptoms and signs consistent with a depressive disorder, and/or associated with distress or dysfunction.

The severity or the duration of the low mood may be out of proportion to the stress that is thought to be causing it. There is no getting around the fact that this incongruity is a subjective determination. But seasoned clinicians can rely on their experiences with other patients in similar circumstances to arrive at a reasonable initial working diagnosis. The situation is easier when there is no discernible stress, that is, when the dysphoric mood appears to occur unexpectedly and manifestly independent of any provocation, because then the dysphoria is clearly unwarranted. (A patient may be unaware of an inciting cause. A discussion of unconscious dynamics is beyond the scope of this article.)

A more objective way to assess abnormality is to look for symptoms and signs that go along with the dejected mood; the existence of a constellation of various features argues that the mood state is abnormal. The features required for the diagnosis of a major depressive episode according to the DSM-IV-TR are listed in **Box 1** and can be recalled using the mnemonic SIG: E CAPS (a prescription for energy capsules). However, even this method is not completely specific because if one labors under an extreme emotional burden, sleep, appetite, and other functions can be disturbed.[6] The situation is further complicated when physical problems cause symptoms consistent with MDD, which are discussed below.

Most clinicians agree that if the low mood causes distress or social or occupational dysfunction, a disorder is present. The DSM-IV-TR requires this feature for the diagnosis of MDD to be made.

Box 1
Criteria for major depressive episode (recalled by the mnemonic SIG: E CAPS)

Symptoms (at least 5 are required, one must be depressed mood or anhedonia)

Depressed mood

Sleep (increased or decreased)

Interest (decreased [anhedonia])

Guilt or feelings of worthlessness

Energy (decreased)

Concentration (decreased)

Appetite (increased or decreased)

Psychomotor agitation or retardation

Suicidal thinking, an attempt, or a plan

Duration

Most of the day, nearly every day, for at least 2 weeks

Severity

Clinically significant distress or functional impairment

Exclusions

Not caused by a medical condition, a substance, or bereavement

Data from American Psychiatric Association. Diagnostic and Statistical Manual of Mental Disorders. Text revision. 4th edition. Washington, DC: American Psychiatric Association; 2000.

Differential Diagnosis of an Abnormal Dysphoric Mood

Once the clinician is convinced that the mood is dysphoric and abnormal (now the term depressed can be used), a consideration of the vast medical and psychiatric differential for depression commences. The various conditions can be grouped into several categories.

Depression may be caused by direct anatomic or physiologic effects of a medical condition (eg, stroke, hypothyroidism) or by the treatment of medical conditions (eg, interferon, corticosteroids). It is important to make a distinction between these secondary depressions and those that might be considered idiopathic (eg, MDD) to tailor treatment and to inform and educate patients properly. For example, hypothyroid patients may be able to discontinue an antidepressant after their thyroid supplementation is adequate.

Depression may be caused by substances of abuse (eg, alcohol, heroin). When evaluating depressive symptoms in a patient who is actively using substances and/or has a long history of substance use, a period of abstinence should be identified and the appraisal of affective symptoms should be confined to that period of sobriety. Such a procedure helps disentangle depressive symptoms due to the substance from those that may be caused by a primary depression. In the authors' experience, it is more often found that patients actually do not feel depressed during such sober periods; only when patients are actively using substances do they meet the criteria for depression. Such a finding is consistent with a substance-induced depressive disorder. Whether or not to use antidepressants in such patients is controversial. Such a procedural approach and diagnostic considerations also apply to substance-related mania or hypomania.

Depression may be caused by a psychological reaction to a medical illness or to its treatment. The depression is not caused by the inherent anatomic or physiologic effects of the medical pathology (as in the category mentioned earlier) but by an emotional response to the stress caused by that pathology (of course, both can occur simultaneously). For example, a devastating illness or injury is often felt as a loss not only of physical well-being but also of autonomy, independence, and self-esteem. Such a loss is then grieved, which is normal. However, grief can sometimes spiral into an adjustment disorder with depressed mood or, if more severe, a full-blown depression; both are abnormal and can, and should, be distinguished from normal grief.

The person who becomes depressed as a result of the psychological stress of a medical illness is to be differentiated from the person who says "I've been depressed my whole life" or some similar statement. Such a declaration should raise suspicion for a fundamental problem in the way individuals negotiate their world, both external and internal. Such persons' depression, as they call it, is not a distinct period of disquietude but a pervasive persistent approach and response to life. More often than not, this characteristic pattern forms the nucleus of a personality disturbance that is best managed by a psychotherapist.

Other psychiatric differential diagnoses of depressed mood include dysthymia (a low-grade depressive state of at least 2 years' duration) and bipolar and schizoaffective disorders (both discussed later).

MDD

A patient who complains of severe depressed mood accompanied by many of the symptoms listed in **Box 1** should look depressed. That is, the examination should accord with the history. The temptation to diagnose MDD simply because the patient meets the criteria should be resisted.[8] In this regard, it is wise to refer to the infrequently read introduction in the DSM-IV-TR, "The specific diagnostic criteria included in DSM-IV are meant to serve as guidelines to be *informed by clinical judgment* and are not meant to be used in a cookbook fashion" (emphasis added).[2(pxxxii)]

Suspicion arises when a patient who is medically ill presents with MDD because several symptoms of MDD are physical and can be caused by somatic illness. There are 3 approaches to this situation: (1) include all symptoms regardless of the presumed cause, (2) exclude the somatic symptoms, and (3) substitute the somatic symptoms with alternative criteria. The authors recommend an approach based on the one used by Chochinov and colleagues,[9] wherein the 2 cardinal criteria of MDD (ie, depressed mood and anhedonia) and the time requirement (most of the day, nearly every day) are applied strictly. The authors place less of a premium on the 2-week requirement and instead are more inclined to diagnose MDD when the patient is clearly suffering or when rehabilitative progress is impeded by depressive symptoms.

APPROACH TO THE PATIENT WITH SUSPECTED BIPOLAR DISORDER

Suspicions of bipolar disorder are raised when patients demonstrate or report major alterations in their usual mood state or behavior. Unfortunately, the protean nature of bipolar disorder is exceeded only by the variable ways that patients, and clinicians, interpret and diagnose it. Debate swirls over whether bipolar disorder is over- or under-diagnosed.[10,11] Rapid cycling, ultrarapid cycling, and expanded subtyping based on "soft signs" are controversial.[12,13] The authors' discussion avoids these debates and controversies and adheres to standard, if not common, practice. The authors recommend that diagnostic ambiguity or controversy calls for conservative practice and, failing that, psychiatric consultation.

Misconceptions about Bipolar Disorder

According to DSM-IV-TR, the defining feature of bipolar disorder is the presence or a history of a manic or a hypomanic episode, the core elements of which can be remembered with the mnemonic DIG FAST (**Box 2**). Recall of such an episode can be quite inaccurate.[14] On the one hand, this inaccuracy means that clinicians must always be alert to the possibility of undiagnosed bipolar disorder, particularly in patients being treated for presumed unipolar depressive illnesses. On the other hand, it provides fertile ground for misinterpretation of both pathologic and ordinary human experiences.

A potentially flawed assessment of bipolarity begins when mania is equated with elation. Excessive happiness is neither necessary nor sufficient for the diagnosis of a manic or hypomanic episode, which should never be framed simply as the emotional opposite of depression. Many manic or hypomanic patients actually experience dysphoria as a prominent mood state.[15] Anger and irritability can be hallmarks of the experience, and intense mood variability is the rule. Lability in the context of a manic episode notwithstanding, bipolar disorder is generally not an explanation for chronic mercurial temperament or a mood that has an irregularly irregular rhythm (ie, varying wildly from moment to moment).

Although patients with bipolar disorder might achieve a stable emotional baseline only infrequently, a solid diagnosis should still document discrete episodes of illness. The authors, while acknowledging the difficulty of retrospective screening for bipolar disorder, favor questions that ask first about a period of at least 4 *consecutive* days with diminished sleep and then about what the patient's energy level was on day 4 or 5. Endorsement of preserved or elevated energy at that point can be followed with purposely vague inquiry into any changes in the patient's thought or behavior

---

Box 2
Criteria for manic and hypomanic episodes (recalled by the mnemonic DIG FAST)

Mood

Abnormally and persistently elevated, expansive, or irritable

Other features (at least 3 are required and at least 4 if mood is irritable)

Distractibility

Indiscretions (eg, shopping sprees, dangerous sexual activities)

Grandiosity

Fast thoughts or flight of ideas

Activity: increase in goal-directed activity

Sleep: decrease in the need for sleep

Talkativeness or pressured (ie, not interruptible) speech

Duration

For mania: one week (or less if hospitalization required)

For hypomania: at least 4 days

Severity

For mania: marked functional or social impairment, or need for hospitalization, or psychosis

For hypomania: unequivocal and observable change in usual functioning

Exclusions

Not caused by a medical condition or a substance

Data from the American Psychiatric Association. Diagnostic and Statistical Manual of Mental Disorders. Text revision. 4th edition. Washington, DC: American Psychiatric Association; 2000.

---

patterns at the time. If the patient spontaneously indicates heightened thought/speech velocity or behavioral impulsivity, one might then ask about the most dramatic example of such an episode that the patient can recall. Only once this semi–open-ended history is obtained should more specific, and unavoidably suggestive, criterion-based questioning be carried out.

Assessment of Dysregulated Mood

The first step in the evaluation of a patient with acutely dysregulated mood or behavior is to determine if the current presentation is best explained by mania or hypomania or by something else. Patients with hyperactive delirium can manifest striking sleep-wake cycle disruption, mood lability, distractibility, disinhibited or aggressive behavior, and frank psychosis.[16] Although at any given moment these patients may cross-sectionally appear manic, delirious patients are distinguished from those with mania by an abrupt onset of the disturbance, a somatic cause, and a fluctuation of consciousness and cognition. This fluctuation cannot be emphasized enough. The only psychopathological states marked by fluctuating consciousness and cognition are delirium, catatonia, and Lewy body dementia.

A dramatic state of hyperactivity and disorganization can precede or be admixed with the more classic vegetative form of catatonia.[17] This hyperactive state overlaps greatly, perhaps entirely, with what some investigators call delirious mania.[18] Although not foolproof, an electroencephalogram can assist in discriminating among mania, delirium, and catatonia.[19] Mania will be marked by a normal alpha (8–12 Hz) rhythm, delirium by diffuse slowing (1–7 Hz), and catatonia by whatever waveform/frequency characterizes its underlying cause (eg, a normal rhythm in primary bipolar, depressive, and psychotic disorders; or epileptiform activity in complex partial seizures).

Demented patients may appear manic or hypomanic because of sleep disturbance, distractibility, disinhibition, and psychosis. The late onset, chronic-progressive nature, and impure (ie, not confined to mania) quality of the psychological signs of dementia are less consistent with mania or hypomania. Patients with frontotemporal dementia, especially Pick disease, present a special challenge because their illness can manifest at an earlier age and with disinhibited behavior rather than with immediately apparent cognitive deficits. Still, the typical presentation of frontotemporal dementia in the sixth decade is quite unusual for primary bipolar illness. Patients with human immunodeficiency virus (HIV) infection, Parkinson disease, and other causes of subcortical dementia also may present with disinhibited behavior. Longitudinal history indicating a chronic-progressive course and so-called frontal lobe dysfunction (eg, deficits in attention, sequencing, planning, or set-shifting) can help to discriminate between incipient dementia and mania or hypomania in these patients.

Primary psychotic disorders (eg, schizophrenia) share bipolar disorder's late adolescent–early adulthood age of onset. Disorganized thinking, self-referential delusions, and impulsive behavior can overlap with manic symptomatology. Exacerbations of psychotic disorders can sometimes be distinguished from mania by the presence of negative symptoms (eg, blunted affect, disinterest, paucity of thought) that are the antitheses of the intense mood and motivational state of the manic patient. The absence of sustained sleeplessness with concomitant preserved or elevated energy also argues against acute mania. Longitudinal history is invaluable in distinguishing mania, which is by definition episodic, from a chronic psychotic condition. Psychotic disorders can be rendered episodic by treatment and compliance factors. In addition, patients with bipolar disorder spend large portions of their lives in depressive states that are not always easily discriminated from negative symptoms.[20] A caveat to the preceding contrasts is schizoaffective disorder, in which episodes of true mania can be intrinsic to the diagnosis (discussed later).

In patients with attention-deficit/hyperactivity disorder (ADHD), restlessness, impulsivity, and high but unproductive activity levels, in conjunction with frequent irritability, relational problems, and sleep disturbances, can be indistinguishable from hypomania or baseline hyperthymia in patients with bipolar II disorder. A similar problem confounds the differential between these states and cluster B personality disorders.[21,22] Comprised of antisocial, narcissistic, histrionic, and borderline personality disorders, cluster B pathologies are defined, among other things, by emotional lability, behavioral impulsivity, and stormy interpersonal relationships. The characteristic episodic course of mania or hypomania can, again, be of help here; however, both ADHD[23] and cluster B personality disorders[24] can coexist with bipolar disorder. As easy as it is to overdiagnose psychiatric comorbidity, there is also no vaccine against other psychiatric dysfunctions coexisting with mania or hypomania. Ongoing assessment, cautious pharmacotherapy, and psychiatric consultation are often necessary in these situations.

Differential Diagnosis of Mania and Hypomania

Once the clinician has determined that a patient's presentation is consistent with a manic or hypomanic episode, that syndrome must be placed in the appropriate diagnostic context. The differential diagnosis of a manic or hypomanic episode extends quite broadly beyond bipolar disorder. The following discussion does not exhaustively cover this differential but provides prototypical diagnostic examples within the critical categories that must be addressed.

A manic or hypomanic episode may result from drug use. Stimulant drugs, including cocaine and amphetamines, are the best-known offenders. Although substance abuse and dependence are well established as very frequently comorbid in bipolar disorder,[25] it can be hard to conclude the independent existence of bipolar disorder without documented evidence of at least one spontaneous (ie, not substance-related) manic or hypomanic episode.

A substance-induced manic or hypomanic episode need not be triggered by illicit substances. Although the degree of risk is unsettled,[26] the use of antidepressants can occasionally precipitate mania or hypomania in patients with known or occult bipolar disorder as well as in some who might never manifest it spontaneously. Nonpsychiatric therapies also may trigger mania or hypomania; corticosteroids are the most notorious example. A handy, but far from inviolate, rule of thumb is that 30 mg of prednisone (or its equivalent) is considered a threshold daily dose for elevated risk of psychiatrically significant symptoms.

Somatic diseases that might cause secondary mania or hypomania are vital to consider in patients with unusual duration, age of onset, or somatic accompaniments to their affective presentation. Examples worth noting as "non-zebras," if not exactly "horses," include hyperthyroidism, Cushing disease, systemic lupus erythematosus, and HIV infection. Just about any infectious, neoplastic, or ischemic brain disease can potentially produce manic or hypomanic symptoms. Acute infectious processes are less likely to produce isolated mania or hypomania in the absence of other neurologic or systemic signs. Neoplastic and ischemic pathologic conditions of the brain are less likely to produce episodic symptoms. The neuroanatomy underlying these processes may involve the temporal lobe and the subcortical structures of the nondominant hemisphere and/or the orbitofrontal cortex.[27] This sort of focality remains vague, and from the authors' observation, there is a fine line between mania and hypomania and the frontal lobe disinhibition syndrome.

Schizoaffective disorder entails criteria similar to those of schizophrenia, joined by the presence of mood episodes for a "substantial portion" of the illness. If one or more of these episodes have been a manic or a mixed (ie, criteria for both mania and depression are simultaneously satisfied) one, then the patient is diagnosed with schizoaffective disorder, bipolar type.

If a manic or a mixed episode has occurred and is not better explained by the alternative possibilities already discussed, then bipolar I disorder is the correct diagnosis. A bipolar II disorder hinges on the occurrence of at least one *hypo*manic episode, plus at least one major depressive episode. Manic or mixed episodes do not occur in bipolar II disorder. Seldom clinically invoked, cyclothymic disorder entails hypomania and subsyndromal depressive symptoms that dominate the patient's affective state for at least a 2-year period with no more than 2 consecutive symptom-free months at a time.

SUMMARY

The first order of business in accurately diagnosing MDD and bipolar disorder is, like everywhere else in medicine, careful history-taking and examination. When dealing with psychiatric symptoms, fastidious use of terminology is especially crucial because the same technical words used by psychiatrists are used also by laymen in their everyday language (eg, depressed, paranoid). Thus it can be easy to assume that both parties mean the same thing when they use the same word. This assumption must be resisted and instead patients must be invited to describe their experiences without using jargon. Likewise, clinicians must neither assume that all sadness is abnormal or caused by MDD nor equate mood swings with bipolar disorder. The mental status examination should accord with the history; if it does not, one needs to revisit the working diagnosis and seek out more information.

REFERENCES

1. Kessler RC, Chiu WT, Demler O, et al. Prevalence, severity, and comorbidity of 12-month DSM-IV disorders in the National Comorbidity Survey Replication. Arch Gen Psychiatry 2005;62:617–27.
2. Wang PS, Lane M, Olfson M, et al. Twelve-month use of mental health services in the United States: results from the National Comorbidity Survey Replication. Arch Gen Psychiatry 2005;62:629–40.
3. Marin RS. Apathy: a neuropsychiatric syndrome. J Neuropsychiatry Clin Neurosci 1991;3:243–54.
4. Slavney PR. Diagnosing demoralization in consultation psychiatry. Psychosomatics 1999;40:325–9.
5. American Psychiatric Association. Diagnostic and statistical manual of mental disorders. Text revision. 4th edition. Washington, DC: American Psychiatric Association; 2000.
6. Horwitz AV, Wakefield JC. The loss of sadness: how psychiatry transformed normal sorrow into depressive disorder. New York: Oxford University Press; 2007.
7. Wakefield JC, Schmitz MF, First MB, et al. Extending the bereavement exclusion for major depression to other losses: evidence from the National Comorbidity Survey. Arch Gen Psychiatry 2007;64:433–40.
8. Kontos N, Freudenreich O, Querques J. Thoughtful diagnoses: not 'checklist' psychiatry. Curr Psychiatr 2007;6:112.
9. Chochinov HM, Wilson KG, Enns M, et al. Prevalence of depression in the terminally ill: effects of diagnostic criteria and symptom threshold judgments. Am J Psychiatry 1994;151:537–40.
10. Smith DJ, Ghaemi N. Is underdiagnosis the main pitfall when diagnosing bipolar disorder? Yes. BMJ 2010;340:854.
11. Zimmerman M. Is underdiagnosis the main pitfall when diagnosing bipolar disorder? No. BMJ 2010;340:855.
12. Bauer M, Beaulieu S, Dunner DL, et al. Rapid cycling bipolar disorder—diagnostic concepts. Bipolar Disord 2008;10:153–62.
13. Akiskal HS. Validating 'hard' and 'soft' phenotypes within the bipolar spectrum: continuity or discontinuity? J Affect Disord 2003;73:1–5.
14. Ruggero CJ, Carlson GA, Kotov R, et al. Ten-year diagnostic consistency of bipolar disorder in a first-admission sample. Bipolar Disord 2010;12:21–31.
15. Goodwin FK, Jamison KR. Manic-depressive illness. New York: Oxford University Press; 1990.
16. Meagher D, Moran M, Raju B, et al. A new data-based motor subtype schema for delirium. J Neuropsychiatry Clin Neurosci 2008;20:185–93.
17. Fricchione GL, Huffman JC, Bush G, et al. Catatonia, neuroleptic malignant syndrome, and serotonin syndrome. In: Stern TA, Rosenbaum JF, Fava M, et al, editors. Massachusetts general hospital comprehensive clinical psychiatry. Philadelphia: Mosby Elsevier; 2008. p. 761–71.
18. Karmacharya R, England ML, Ongur D. Delirious mania: clinical features and treatment response. J Affect Disord 2008;109:312–6.

19. Jacobson S, Jerrier H. EEG in delirium. Semin Clin Neuropsychiatry 2000;5: 86–92.

20. Judd LL, Akiskal HS, Schettler PJ, et al. The long-term natural history of the weekly symptomatic status of bipolar I disorder. Arch Gen Psychiatry 2002;59: 530–7.

21. Zimmerman M, Ruggero CJ, Chelminski I, et al. Psychiatric diagnoses in patients previously diagnosed with bipolar disorder. J Clin Psychiatry 2010;71:26–31.

22. Janowsky DS, Leff M, Epstein RS. Playing the manic game. Arch Gen Psychiatry 1970;22:252–61.

23. Klassen LJ, Katzman MA, Chokka P. Adult ADHD and its comorbidities, with a focus on bipolar disorder. J Affect Disord 2010;124:1–8.

24. Fan AH, Hassell J. Bipolar disorder and comorbid personality psychopathology. J Clin Psychiatry 2008;69:1794–803.

25. Strakowski SM, DelBello MP, Fleck DE, et al. The impact of substance abuse on the course of bipolar disorder. Biol Psychiatry 2000;48:477–85.

26. Goldberg JF. Antidepressants in bipolar disorder: 7 myths and realities. Curr Psychiatr 2010;9:40–9.

27. Starkstein SE, Manes F. Manic and manic-like disorders. In: Bogusslavsky J, Cummings JL, editors. Behavior and mood disorders in focal brain lesions. New York: Cambridge University Press; 2000. p. 202–16.

An Approach to the Patient with Anxiety

Daniel Hicks, MD, Thomas Cummings Jr, MD,
Steven A. Epstein, MD*

KEYWORDS

• Anxiety disorders • Primary care • Panic disorder
• Generalized anxiety disorder • Anxiolytics

EPIDEMIOLOGY

According to the National Comorbidity Survey Replication (NCS-R), anxiety disorders are the most common psychiatric disorders in the general population; the 12-month and lifetime incidence are 19% and 31%, respectively. Among anxiety disorders, generalized anxiety disorder (GAD), panic disorder (PD), post-traumatic stress disorder (PTSD), social anxiety disorder (SAD), and specific phobia are the most prevalent. The NCS-R data also confirm that anxiety disorders are roughly twice as common in women as they are in men and that they frequently co-occur.[1,2]

The prevalence of anxiety disorders (GAD, PD, PTSD, and social phobia) in the primary care setting is similar to that in the general population.[3] Accordingly, approximately 48% of all visits for symptoms of anxiety are to primary care physicians (PCPs)[4]; frequently, anxiety occurs in those with chronic medical conditions, such as arthritis, heart disease, gastrointestinal [GI] disease, and hypertension.[5] Although specific phobias are the most common anxiety disorder, they rarely precipitate primary care visits.

Direct and indirect costs of anxiety disorders in the United States total $40 billion annually.[4] Kroenke and colleagues[3] confirmed that anxiety disorders in the primary care setting are associated with impaired function in social domains and work, poorer general health and higher pain levels, and more physician visits and disability days used. Anxiety may increase the risk of medical illnesses (eg, angina, arrhythmias, labile hypertension, irritable bowel syndrome [IBS]) and exacerbate them. Anxiety may also lead to coronary artery disease (CAD),[6] hypertension,[7] and cardiovascular morbidity.[7,8]

Currently, the *Diagnostic and Statistical Manual of Mental Disorders, Fifth Edition's* proposed revisions include a new disorder termed mixed anxiety depression,[9] a common diagnosis in countries outside the United States.

Department of Psychiatry, Georgetown University Hospital and School of Medicine, Street–2115 Wisconsin Avenue, Suite 200, Washington, DC 20007, USA
* Corresponding author.
E-mail address: epsteins@gunet.georgetown.edu

Med Clin N Am 94 (2010) 1127–1139
doi:10.1016/j.mcna.2010.08.008
0025-7125/10/$ – see front matter © 2010 Elsevier Inc. All rights reserved.

PATHOPHYSIOLOGY

Abnormalities in the neural circuitry (within the amygdala, medial prefrontal cortex, insular cortex, and hippocampus) underlie fear, memory, and emotions; specifically, PD, PTSD, and social phobia are associated with a hyperresponsive amygdala and a hyporesponsive medial prefrontal cortex.[10]

On the neurochemical level, norepinephrine (NE), serotonin (5-HT), and γ-aminobutyric acid (GABA) are thought to play a significant role in anxiety disorders (eg, with under-activation of serotonergic function, complex dysregulation and overactivation of noradrenergic function). Further, decreased $GABA_A$ and $5-HT_{1A}$ receptor binding in the limbic system have been found in those with PD,[11,12] consistent with the data on pharmaceutical therapies that target 5-HT, NE, and GABA systems.

DIAGNOSIS AND CLASSIFICATION

Because of underreporting by patients and under-recognition by physicians, anxiety disorders often go unrecognized in the primary care setting.

The hallmarks of GAD are excessive worry, difficulty contrclling the worry, and several physical (eg, fatigue, muscle tension) and psychological (eg, irritability, poor concentration) symptoms that have lasted at least 6 months; frequently, sufferers are chronically anxious and have been called "worriers."[13] Somatic symptoms and insomnia are typically reported to the internist.

PD is characterized by recurrent panic attacks (episodes of intense anxiety), significant physical distress (eg, palpitations, sweating, tremulousness, shortness of breath, chest pain, fear of choking, dizziness, and fear of dying or losing control), and anxiety about having another panic attack.[13]

At least one-third of individuals with chest pain and normal coronary arteries have PD.[14] Correlates of PD include absence of CAD, atypical quality of chest pain, female gender; younger age, and self-reported anxiety.[15]

Patients with benign palpitations are also prone to PD[16]; however, they should undergo a cardiac evaluation (eg, with ambulatory electrocardiographic monitoring) to rule-out arrhythmias. Although PD and mitral valve prolapse were linked for many years, data do not support a clear relationship.[17] Patients with PD commonly suffer from medical symptoms and conditions, eg, dizziness[18] and IBS.[19]

PTSD stems from exposure to a traumatic event (eg, a military experience, a physical or sexual assault, a motor vehicle accident, a natural disaster) that involved actual or threatened death or serious injury to oneself or others resulting in fear, helplessness, or horror. Symptoms of PTSD last longer than one month and are classified as re-experiencing (eg, distressing recollections of the trauma with illusions and hallucinations, intense physiologic responses when presented with exposure cues related to the traumatic event, nightmares), avoidance and numbing, and increased arousal (eg, hypervigilance, exaggerated startle response, insomnia, irritability, poor concentration).[13] PTSD symptoms are particularly common among survivors of acute trauma (eg, burns,[20] motor vehicle accidents).[21]

SAD is marked by a pronounced fear of social or performance situations; afflicted individuals fear that they will do something embarrassing, which causes distress, impaired function, and avoidance of certain situations.[13]

Obsessive-compulsive disorder (OCD) is defined by the presence of distressing, time-consuming, and impairing and intrusive obsessions (thoughts, images, or impulses) or compulsions (repetitive behaviors or mental acts performed in response to an obsession) intended to reduce distress or prevent a dreaded event. Patients with

OCD recognize that their obsessions (eg, an unrealistic fear of germs) and compulsions (eg, repetitive hand-washing) are excessive or unreasonable.[13]

SCREENING AND EVALUATION

Although primarily directed at screening for GAD, the GAD 7-item scale (GAD-7) is highly sensitive to and specific for other anxiety disorders (eg, PD, SAD, and PTSD).[3,22] The GAD-7 (**Fig. 1**) may be completed quickly and easily in the primary care setting, and it serves as a useful tool for screening. It is a self-report measure that provides a probable diagnosis that may then be confirmed by an interview. It also is an excellent measure for monitoring response to treatment. A score of 8 or greater is highly suggestive of an anxiety disorder, and a total score of 10 or greater indicates a probable diagnosis of GAD. The first 2 items represent an even briefer scale called the GAD-2; a score of 3 or greater is significantly associated with the most common anxiety disorders.

CAUSES OF ANXIETY

Predisposing factors (eg, childhood stressors and a family history of anxiety) are common. Nonetheless, considering potential precipitating factors for every patient is important. Causes of anxiety include a psychological reaction to having a medical

Over the <u>last 2 weeks</u> , how often have you been bothered by the following problems? *(Use "☐" to indicate your answer)*	Not at all	Several days	More than half the days	Nearly every day
1. Feeling nervous, anxious or on edge	0	1	2	3
2. Not being able to stop or control worrying	0	1	2	3
3. Worrying too much about different things	0	1	2	3
4. Trouble relaxing	0	1	2	3
5. Being so restless that it is hard to sit still	0	1	2	3
6. Becoming easily annoyed or irritable	0	1	2	3
7. Feeling afraid as if something awful might happen	0	1	2	3

(For office coding: Total Score T_____ = ___ + ___ + ___)

Fig. 1. GAD-7. Copyright © 2005 Pfizer, Inc. All rights reserved.

illness or another life stressor, the direct effect of a substance or of substance withdrawal, and the biologic effects of a medical illness.

When faced with life stressors (eg, medical illness), individuals prone to anxiety become anxious.[23,24] Even routine evaluations cause anxiety, especially among those with a personal or family history of illness (eg, breast cancer) who might become anxious before routine testing (eg, mammography). Anxiety may also arise between the initial evaluation and receiving the definitive diagnosis. Prolonged diagnostic uncertainty becomes even more anxiety-provoking.

Uncertainty Regarding Medical Prognosis

Many patients experience episodic fear, especially when illness has a tendency to recur (eg, arrhythmias, cancer, multiple sclerosis). Even those who have favorable prognoses often become anxious. For example, a 95% cure rate is reassuring to most patients, but some have difficulty coping with the prospect of a 5% recurrence rate. For patients who learn about their prognosis through personal medical searches, physicians may be able to provide reassurance by telling the anxious patient: "Those data were published before the newest treatments became available."

Anxiety About One's Body

Many individuals develop anxiety regarding future effects of their illness (eg, amputation from complications of diabetes mellitus and peripheral vascular disease), loss of functional capacity (eg, blindness), or becoming overly dependent on others; knowledge of these fears can help the physician provide appropriate reassurance (eg, that pain will be aggressively treated).

Fear of Death

Almost all individuals, regardless of their physical health, fear death at some point. Physicians must be comfortable assessing fear of death in patients and their families. This assessment must include an exploration of specific reasons for a fear of death. Exploration of the reasons for an irrational estimate of the risk of death may lead to straightforward reassurance or discover another issue (eg, patients may be afraid that their family would not be able to survive without them).

Anxiety About the Impact of Illness on Identity and Livelihood

Even if illness is insufficient to cause anxiety, patients may be concerned about their ability to work, perform essential household functions, pay for treatment, or maintain income. The uninsured or underinsured are often so anxious about how they would pay for medical procedures that they avoid medical visits altogether. In these situations, meetings with family members and health care financial counselors may help to assuage unjustifiable fears.

Anxiety Regarding Strangers and Being Alone in the Hospital

Some individuals become anxious even when their own personal physician performs a medical procedure. Thus, it is understandable that intense anxiety arises when being treated by a new physician in the emergency department or intensive care unit. Others (with dependency needs) regress in the hospital and become unduly anxious when left alone in an unfamiliar environment.

Anxiety Regarding Negative Reactions from Physicians

Some individuals worry about their physician's opinion of them. Excessive concern may lead to reluctance to seek health care. People who feel guilty for not following their physician's recommendations might cancel appointments for fear of being scolded (eg, for failure to lose weight, stop smoking, or check blood sugar levels more reliably). Similarly, some individuals have anxiety that might lead them to fail to disclose important information (eg, regarding sexual risk factors or level of alcohol intake). Consistent and firm reminders of the need for proper medical care are warranted and may contribute to enhanced adherence.

Substance-Induced Anxiety

Before evaluating whether medications may cause anxiety, it is important to assess whether the patient's anxiety may be due to withdrawal from substances of abuse (eg, alcohol, sedative-hypnotics, anxiolytics).[13] Patients may be reluctant to disclose such information or may minimize the severity of the problem; collateral history, for example, from family members, is often essential.

Caffeine and over-the-counter (OTC) sympathomimetics are common causes of anxiety. Caffeine may be present in significant quantities in coffee, tea, caffeinated soda, caffeinated water, herbal preparations (eg, Ephedra), and coffee ice cream, as well as in OTC preparations for alertness (eg, Caffeine), weight loss, and headache (eg, Acetaminophen, Aspirin, and Caffeine).[25] In individuals with an anxiety disorder, reduction of caffeine intake often relieves anxiety.

A bevy of medications have been associated with anxiety (eg, angiotensin-converting enzyme inhibitors, β-adrenergic agonists, corticosteroids, estrogens, histamine (H_2) receptor antagonists, interferon, sympathomimetics, prokinetic agents [eg, metoclopramide], and psychostimulants).[26–28]

Anxiety Secondary to General Medical Conditions

Medical problems have also been linked to anxiety, but data are often derived from case reports. It is particularly important to evaluate medical causes of anxiety when the history is not typical of an anxiety disorder (eg, lack of personal or family history, lack of psychosocial stressors) and when the anxiety develops at a later age, when it is accompanied by prominent physical symptoms (eg, marked dyspnea, tachycardia, or tremor), or when there are physical symptoms that do not typically accompany anxiety (eg, syncope, confusion, or focal neurologic symptoms).

The evaluation of an anxious patient should include[29] a history and physical examination, including neurologic examination, an evaluation of the potential role of medications and substances, and screening diagnostic studies (eg, routine blood chemistries, complete blood cell count, calcium concentration, thyroid hormone levels, electrocardiogram); a screening thyroid-stimulating hormone (TSH) level should be obtained for patients with new-onset anxiety disorders and treatment-resistant anxiety, particularly when the anxiety is generalized and accompanied by prominent physical symptoms. If the TSH level is abnormal, further evaluation of the thyroid axis is recommended (eg, a free thyroxine index or free thyroxine measurement).

Anxiety symptoms occur commonly in individuals with both subclinical and clinical hyperthyroidism.[30] Hyperthyroidism (with persistent tachycardia, warm and dry palms, and fatigue accompanied by the desire to be active) may be difficult to distinguish from a primary anxiety disorder.[29] Improvement in anxiety usually parallels successful treatment of the hyperthyroidism. Nonetheless, antianxiety treatment should be considered during normalization of thyroid hormone levels, particularly for individuals with moderate-to-severe symptoms. β-Blockers, used routinely for the acute treatment of hyperthyroidism, also relieve peripheral manifestations of anxiety.

Rates of anxiety disorders among individuals with asthma and chronic obstructive pulmonary disease (COPD) are higher than among those in the general population.[31]

It is essential to consider physiological factors intrinsic to asthma. For example, both hypercapnia and hyperventilation may lead to symptoms of a panic attack.[32] Asthma may also be associated with panic attacks through a process of classical conditioning. In this paradigm, because an asthma attack can be terrifying, a future sensation of mild dyspnea might precipitate a full-blown episode of panic.[33] In addition, anxiety may worsen asthma, contributing to a vicious circle in which pulmonary and anxiety symptoms exacerbate each other.[33] Pulmonary emboli[34] may also lead to anxiety.

Anxiety often appears after the onset of Parkinson's disease.[35,36] For example, some individuals may develop symptoms of SAD, because they are embarrassed about manifestations of the Parkinson's disease (eg, tremor).[13] Depression and anxiety symptoms often co-exist in Parkinson's disease,[37] and anxiety may also be secondary to medications used to treat Parkinson's disease (eg, levodopa).

While poststroke depression has been more widely described, many individuals also develop poststroke anxiety,[37] alone or in combination with depression.[38] When poststroke anxiety appears, it may persist. For example, in one large study, 40% of patients still had anxiety after six months.[37] Such anxiety has been associated with right-hemispheric lesions, whereas depression and mixed depression and anxiety are more commonly associated with left-hemispheric lesions.[39]

Complex partial seizures may also be accompanied by symptoms of PD (eg, fear, depersonalization, derealization, dizziness, paresthesias).[40] Anxiety may be associated with hypocalcemia and hypomagnesemia. Relatively rare conditions for which there are only limited data supporting a causal relationship include carcinoid syndrome, hyperparathyroidism, and pheochromocytoma.[29]

TREATMENT

Once the diagnosis of an anxiety disorder has been made, several safe and effective treatment options are available; unfortunately, only about 25% of patients receive an adequate trial of medication, and even fewer receive appropriate counseling.[41] Almost half the patients with an anxiety disorder screened in primary care clinics receive no treatment.[42] Effective treatment can decrease anxiety symptoms and comorbid somatic symptoms and lead to improved health and quality of life; it may involve the use of medications, psychotherapy, or both. Response rates to medications are highest for PD (up to 70%) and lowest for OCD (as low as 50%).[43] Cognitive-behavioral psychotherapy (CBT) has comparable efficacy, and a combination of medication and psychotherapy may lead to even higher rates of improvement.[44]

PHARMACOLOGIC TREATMENTS
Antidepressants

Selective serotonin reuptake inhibitors (SSRIs) and serotonin norepinephrine reuptake inhibitors (SNRIs) are generally considered the most effective medications for anxiety disorders. SSRIs increase the availability of 5-HT, which is thought to be reduced in anxiety disorders. SNRIs also increase NE, which is involved in the regulation of fear-conditioning and stress-response. All SSRIs are thought to be equally effective, but they differ in their side-effect profiles. Because they inhibit cytochrome P450 2D6, fluoxetine and paroxetine can cause significant drug interactions; they are often avoided in persons on multiple medications; sertraline, citalopram, and escitalopram are preferentially used in the medically ill. In elderly and medically ill patients or those with known sensitivity to medications, it is best to begin at a lower dose, then gradually increase to a therapeutic dose (when accommodation to early side effects has occurred). Common side effects of SSRIs and SNRIs (eg, nausea and GI symptoms, sexual dysfunction, sedation, activation) are mild and tend to subside after a few days (except for sexual side effects). Early activation may lead to exacerbation of anxiety. Blood pressure elevation may develop with the use of SNRIs and may necessitate discontinuation.

All SSRIs and SNRIs take at least 3 to 4 weeks to achieve full effect; when only partially effective, the dosage should be increased every 3 to 4 weeks until the maximal recommended dosage is reached or limited side effects are encountered. Patients should generally stay on the medication for 6 to 8 weeks at a maximal dose before the medication is determined to be ineffective. At that point, the medication may need to be switched or augmented. For more severe or persistent disorders, especially OCD, higher doses may be needed.[45] Fluvoxamine, an SSRI, is approved only for OCD; because of its inhibition of cytochrome P450 3A4, it can have many drug-drug interactions.

Tricyclic antidepressants (TCAs) and monoamine oxidase inhibitors (MAOIs) are effective for anxiety disorders. However, TCAs cause sedation, dry mouth, constipation, blurred vision, and orthostatic hypotension and can be lethal in overdose because of a quinidinelike effect on the heart. Therefore, they are rarely used as first-line treatments. MAOIs require strict dietary restrictions and avoidance of many medications (including common OTC cold medications), because interactions can cause life-threatening hypertension. Consequently, MAOIs are rarely used unless the patient is very compliant. The new selegiline transdermal patch avoids the need for some of the dietary restrictions, but it is approved only for depression, not for anxiety disorders. The TCA, clomipramine, was approved in this country specifically for treatment of OCD, but because it causes the same problems as other TCAs, it should be used only if other treatments have failed.

Mirtazapine, a unique medication that acts on specific serotoninergic and noradrenergic receptors, tends to be sedating and anxiolytic, but it should be considered as a second-line agent or as an adjunctive treatment with SSRIs.

Benzodiazepines

Benzodiazepines are the most rapid-acting and effective medications used to relieve anxiety. Lorazepam has the advantage of multiple routes of administration, oral, intravenous, or intramuscular, has no active metabolite, and requires only conjugation and, thus, less metabolic effort by the liver.[46] Alprazolam is the best-studied treatment of PD. However, its short half-life and requirement for frequent dosing (to avoid interdose withdrawal) limits its usefulness. The extended-release formulation still usually requires twice-daily dosing and is more expensive.[47] Clonazepam is also approved for the treatment of PD and has the advantage of a longer half-life and less rebound or withdrawal problems. The older benzodiazepines, such as diazepam and chlordiazepoxide, have longer half-lives, which can lead to more sedation and cognitive impairment with accumulation of drug levels.

The disadvantages of using benzodiazepines include sedation, fatigue, motor and cognitive impairment, increased risk of falls (especially in elderly patients), respiratory depression, and risk of accidents due to slowed reaction times. Also, sustained, regular usage leads to physical dependency and to the risk of withdrawal (similar to alcohol withdrawal). For persons at risk of substance abuse or dependence or who are in early recovery, benzodiazepines can lead to addiction. Alcohol should be avoided in persons taking benzodiazepines.

Because of the immediate relief from anxiety that benzodiazepines can bring, they can be helpful and effective, especially for PD and GAD. The best approach is to use them as adjuncts for a few weeks while starting an SSRI or SNRI, after which the benzodiazepine can be tapered off. This should be carefully explained to the patient, because some prefer the immediate relief of the benzodiazepine. Some people with more severe anxiety can be maintained on benzodiazepines, either regularly or as needed. Most of them will have no problems with addiction, although they may become physically dependent and need a slow tapering off to prevent physiologic withdrawal.

Buspirone

Buspirone is a unique anxiolytic that does not cause sedation, dependency, or respiratory depression. It has been found to be somewhat helpful in some persons with GAD but not PD or other anxiety disorders. It may be a good alternative for treatment of GAD in those at risk of substance dependence or for those with COPD or other medical illnesses for which benzodiazepines should be avoided. It may also be useful as an adjunct to other medications, such as SSRIs.

Antipsychotics

The advent of second-generation or atypical antipsychotics, such as quetiapine and risperidone, has led to several studies showing efficacy in treating anxiety disorders; however, none of these agents have been approved for this usage. They are generally not used as first-line agents but may be used for augmentation in refractory anxiety disorders (eg, severe OCD, PTSD, or PD). Because of their higher risk of metabolic and neurologic side effects, they should be used in consultation with psychiatric colleagues. Quetiapine has been used successfully to treat anxiety in patients being weaned off a ventilator, when benzodiazepines may interfere with respiratory drive.[48]

Antihypertensives

β-Blockers, such as propranolol, cause physical symptoms of anxiety (tremor, palpitations, and sweating) but not the anxiety itself. They are usually used for performance anxiety (eg, before public speaking, performing, or test-taking). Some data indicates that propranolol given immediately after an acute trauma may reduce the development of PTSD.[49]

α_2-adrenergic agonists decrease central adrenergic activity and have been proposed for the treatment of PTSD. Prazosin has been shown to reduce nightmares, improve sleep, and reduce hyperarousal, re-experiencing, and numbing.[50]

COUNSELING AND PSYCHOTHERAPY

Once an anxiety disorder is recognized, the first steps in treatment are providing support and information. Patient education about anxiety and how it causes physical symptoms can lead to a its reduction and may help instill a sense of control. General stress reduction measures (eg, regular exercise, sleep hygiene, and avoidance of alcohol, caffeine, nicotine, and other substances) are important. Basic relaxation techniques (eg, deep breathing, progressive muscle relaxation) can also be taught.[47] Self-help manuals and Web sites are available for those who want further information and support, such as the Anxiety Disorders Association of American (www.adaa.org) and the International Obsessive-Compulsive Foundation (www.ocfoundation.org). Most people also benefit from psychotherapy and should be referred to an appropriate mental health professional. Studies have shown that this can be done effectively in the primary care clinic setting.[51]

CBT

CBT has been shown to be the most effective form of psychotherapy for most anxiety disorders. Many individuals prefer psychotherapy to medication, and the two can be combined successfully. For milder cases of anxiety, medications and simple behavioral techniques (eg, sleep hygiene, exercise, and relaxation techniques, such as breath control and progressive muscle relaxation) can be used in the primary care office. Scheduling pleasurable activities, such as taking a walk, or going to a concert or movie also can be helpful for those who are anxious and unable to relax. Distraction techniques, such as listening to soothing music or thinking about a pleasurable memory to replace anxiety-provoking thoughts, can also be effective. Simple cognitive techniques (eg, becoming aware of catastrophic thoughts that lead to anxiety, such as "I know that I will fail." or "Everyone will ridicule me." and replacing them with more rational thoughts) can be a first step in gaining control over the anxiety.

For more difficult cases of anxiety, the patient should be referred to a clinician who is proficient in CBT. It is generally conducted over several weeks and involves psychoeducation about anxiety and its effects, self-monitoring, and grounding techniques, such as relaxation exercises. Cognitive restructuring is done by helping the patient identify thoughts and triggers that can lead to anxiety symptoms, then modifying or changing these thoughts to prevent the symptom. Homework assignments are usually given to help patients practice these techniques and become more conscious of their role in anxiety. The patient is encouraged to develop safety techniques, such as carrying as-needed medication, ensuring a plan to exit if panic ensues, and having access to supportive persons. This type of therapy can be effective either when done individually or in a group.[47]

Exposure and response prevention therapy is especially effective for persons with OCD.[52] In this treatment, the patient is gradually exposed to situations that cause anxiety and then prevented from engaging in compulsive behaviors. For example, a patient with fears of contamination might initially imagine exposure to dirt. Gradually the imaginal events would increase to more intense situations, and the person would be exposed to the actual feared situation while being required to resist the compulsive behavior (eg, hand washing).

CBT can generally be accomplished over a brief period (eg, over 8–12 sessions). Strategies, once learned, can have a long-lasting effect, but sometimes require "booster" sessions to reinforce the learning over time.

Mindfulness therapy is a type of CBT that uses meditation techniques as a way of gaining awareness and control over physical and emotional symptoms. It has been used alone and in conjunction with other therapeutic approaches to reduce stress, anxiety, depression, and pain.[53]

Psychodynamic Psychotherapy

There is less evidence showing the efficacy of psychodynamic psychotherapy for the treatment of anxiety disorders. This therapeutic approach involves exploring the patient's biopsychosocial development and the events before the onset of symptoms, with the goal of understanding the meaning of the anxiety in light of the person's personality and development. Prior coping mechanisms and strengths are then used to help the person develop a sense of mastery and control over the anxiety symptoms. This intervention should be performed by mental health colleagues.

COLLABORATIVE CARE

There is increasing evidence that an effective approach to treating anxiety disorders in primary care involves systematic collaboration of psychiatrists and other mental health clinicians with the primary care practices. In collaborative care, the internist and specially trained care manager provide the mental health treatment, with the psychiatrist serving primarily as a consultant. Care managers can be nurses or office staff in the primary care office or mental health clinicians who work in coordination with the clinic. The medication changes can also be done by the PCPs, with psychiatric consultation used only in more difficult cases. In one study, elderly patients were screened for anxiety disorders in a primary care clinic, then treated with CBT by mental health clinicians over 3 months in the same setting. This intervention led to decreases in worry and depression and improvement in mental health; changes were maintained for up to a year.[51] In another study, a primary care practice incorporated 2 psychiatric visits for evaluation and treatment of patients identified as having PD. Also, follow-up phone calls were made over the course of the year by specially trained care managers to assess symptomatology and side effects and advise medication changes in consultation with the psychiatrist. These patients were much more likely to adhere to treatment and to receive an adequate type, dose, and duration of treatment than those in usual care. Despite the increased cost for the mental health care, the overall cost of care was less, thought to be because of fewer somatic symptoms once the anxiety was treated.[54]

PROGNOSIS

The prognosis of anxiety disorders varies with diagnosis, severity of symptoms, and presence of comorbidities (eg, depression or substance abuse). Once the diagnosis is made, treatment can be effective. In social anxiety, PD, and GAD, response rates are around 80% with medication and psychotherapy.[55] PTSD and OCD are more difficult to treat, with initial response rates of around 50%, but symptoms can be reduced by augmentation with psychotherapy or other medications.[55]

Because anxiety disorders tend to be chronic, if a significant response (>50% improvement) or remission is achieved, medications should be continued for 6 to 12 months and then gradually tapered off. Stopping SSRIs and SNRIs precipitously can cause withdrawal symptoms, and benzodiazepines (especially those with a half-life of 10–20 hours) must be tapered off to avoid a possible life-threatening withdrawal. If symptoms recur, the medications should be maintained longer, especially in more refractory or severe anxiety disorders. Patients can be safely maintained on medications indefinitely if necessary, to keep their symptoms under control. If CBT has been effective, booster sessions can be used to control or decrease symptoms. More severe cases of OCD, PD, or PTSD that have caused serious symptoms or disability may require lifetime medication management and therapy.

SUMMARY

Anxiety disorders are the most common of all psychiatric illnesses, causing significant impairment and distress. Unfortunately, they frequently go unrecognized and undertreated. Most people with anxiety present to PCPs with physical symptoms, such as fatigue, insomnia, pain, dyspnea, headaches, and GI symptoms. Screening for anxiety disorders is essential to diagnose and treat these illnesses. Milder cases of anxiety disorders may be effectively treated in the primary care office with medications and simple CBT techniques. Another developing approach is coordination of care between primary care and mental health practitioners, so that patients can be seen, assessed, and treated in the primary care office by mental health clinicians or by their own staff in consultation with psychiatrists or mental health providers. If the person's symptoms are more severe or do not respond to initial medication trials, they should be referred to a psychiatrist or mental health practitioner for further evaluation and treatment. Access to available mental health clinicians is often limited, because of inadequate mental health coverage by many insurance plans and a dearth of clinicians in certain areas; this problem may be alleviated with the new mental health parity laws and health care reform. As recent studies have shown, integration of mental health services into primary care may be the most effective way to diagnose and treat anxiety disorders and other psychiatric illnesses.

REFERENCES

1. National Comorbidity Survey [internet]. NCS-R appendix tables 1 and 2. Available at: http://www.hcp.med.harvard.edu/ncs/publications.php. Accessed July 19, 2007.
2. Kessler RC, Chiu WT, Demler O, et al. Prevalence, severity, and comorbidity of 12-month DSM-IV disorders in the National Comorbidity Survey Replication. Arch Gen Psychiatry 2005;62:617–27.
3. Kroenke K, Spitzer RL, Williams JB, et al. Anxiety disorders in primary care: prevalence, impairment, comorbidity, and detection. Ann Intern Med 2007;146(5): 317–25.
4. Harman JS, Rollman BL, Hanusa BH, et al. Physician office visits of adults for anxiety disorders in the United States, 1985–1998. J Gen Intern Med 2002;17: 165–72.
5. Sareen J, Jacobi F, Cox BJ, et al. Disability and poor quality of life associated with comorbid anxiety disorders and physical conditions. Arch Intern Med 2006; 166(19):2109–16.
6. Albert CM, Chae CU, Rexrode KM, et al. Phobic anxiety and risk of coronary heart disease and sudden cardiac death among women. Circulation 2005;111:480–7.
7. Jonas BS, Franks P, Ingram DD. Are symptoms of anxiety and depression risk factors for hypertension? Longitudinal evidence from the national health and nutrition examination survey I epidemiologic follow-up study. Arch Fam Med 1997;6:43–9.
8. Smoller JW, Pollack MH, Wassertheil-Smoller S, et al. Panic attacks and risk of incident cardiovascular events among postmenopausal women in the Women's Health Initiative observational study. Arch Gen Psychiatry 2007;64(10):1153–60.
9. Available at: http://dsm5.org. Accessed April 24, 2010.
10. Shin LM, Orr SP, Carson MA, et al. Regional cerebral blood flow in amygdala and medial prefrontal cortex during traumatic imagery in male and female Vietnam veterans with PTSD. Arch Gen Psychiatry 2004;61:168–76.
11. Hasler G, Nugent AC, Carlson PJ, et al. Altered cerebral gamma-aminobutyric acid type A-benzodiazepine receptor binding in panic disorder determined by [11C]flumazenil positron emission tomography. Arch Gen Psychiatry 2008;65: 1166–75.
12. Nash JR, Sargent PA, Rabiner EA, et al. Serotonin 5-HT1A receptor binding in people with panic disorder: positron emission tomography study. Br J Psychiatry 2008;193:229–34.
13. American Psychiatric Association. Diagnostic and statistical manual of mental disorders. text rev. 4th edition. Washington, DC: American Psychiatric Association; 2000.
14. Bringager CB, Friis S, Arnesen H, et al. Nine-year follow-up of panic disorder in chest pain patients: clinical course and predictors of outcome. Gen Hosp Psychiatry 2008;30(2):138–46.
15. Huffman JC, Pollack MH. Predicting panic disorder among patients with chest pain: an analysis of the literature. Psychosomatics 2003;44:222–36.

16. Ehlers A, Mayou RA, Sprigings DC, et al. Psychological and perceptual factors associated with arrhythmias and benign palpitations. Psychosom Med 2000;62:693–702.

17. Filho AS, Maciel BC, Martin-Santos R, et al. Does the association between mitral valve prolapse and panic disorder really exist? Prim Care Companion J Clin Psychiatry 2008;10(1):38–47.

18. Yardley L, Owen N, Nazareth I, et al. Panic disorder with agoraphobia associated with dizziness: characteristic symptoms and psychosocial sequelae. J Nerv Ment Dis 2001;189(5):321–7.

19. Sugaya N, Kaiya H, Kumano H, et al. Relationship between subtypes of irritable bowel syndrome and severity of symptoms associated with panic disorder. Scand J Gastroenterol 2008;43(6):675–81.

20. McKibben JB, Bresnick MG, Wiechman Askay SA, et al. Acute stress disorder and posttraumatic stress disorder: a prospective study of prevalence, course, and predictors in a sample with major burn injuries. J Burn Care Res 2008;29(1):22–35.

21. Zatzick DF, Kang SM, Muller HG, et al. Predicting posttraumatic distress in hospitalized trauma survivors with acute injuries. Am J Psychiatry 2002;159:941–6.

22. Spitzer RL, Kroenke K, Williams JB, et al. A brief measure for assessing generalized anxiety disorder: the GAD-7. Arch Intern Med 2006;166:1092–7.

23. Strain JJ, Grossman S. Psychological care of the medically ill. New York: Appleton-Century-Crofts; 1975.

24. Kahana RJ, Bibring GL. Personality types in medical management. In: Zinberg N, editor. Psychiatry and medical practice in a general hospital. New York: International Universities Press; 1964. p. 108–23.

25. Childs E, Hohoff C, Deckert J, et al. Association between ADORA2A and DRD2 polymorphisms and caffeine-induced anxiety. Neuropsychopharmacology 2008;33(12):2791–800.

26. Drugs that may cause psychiatric symptoms, in The medical letter on drugs and therapeutics. 2008.

27. Epstein SA, Hicks DA. Anxiety disorders. In: Levenson JL, editor. Textbook of psychosomatic medicine. 2nd edition, in press.

28. Physicians' desk reference. Montvale (NJ): Thomson Reuters; 2009.

29. Colon EA, Popkin MK. Anxiety and panic. In: Wise MG, Rundell JR, editors. The american psychiatric publishing textbook of consultation-liaison psychiatry. 2nd edition. Washington, DC: American Psychiatric Publishing; 2002. p. 393–415.

30. Gulseren S, Gulseren L, Hekimsoy Z, et al. Depression, anxiety, health-related quality of life, and disability in patients with overt and subclinical thyroid dysfunction. Arch Med Res 2006;37(1):133–9.

31. Hasler G, Gergen PJ, Kleinbaum DG, et al. Asthma and panic in young adults: a 20-year prospective community study. Am J Respir Crit Care Med 2005; 171(11):1224–30.

32. Zaubler TS, Katon W. Panic disorder in the general medical setting. J Psychosom Res 1998;44:25–42.

33. Deshmukh VM, Toelle BG, Usherwood T, et al. The association of comorbid anxiety and depression with asthma-related quality of life and symptom perception in adults. Respirology 2008;13(5):695–702.

34. Tapson VF. Pulmonary embolism. In: Goldman L, Ausiello D, editors. Cecil textbook of medicine. 23rd edition. Philadelphia: WB Saunders; 2007. p. 688–95. Chapter 99.

35. Pontone GM, Williams JR, Anderson KE, et al. Prevalence of anxiety disorders and anxiety subtypes in patients with Parkinson's disease. Mov Disord 2009; 24(9):1333–8.

36. Richard IH. Anxiety disorders in Parkinson's disease. Adv Neurol 2005;96:42–55.
37. De Wit L, Putman K, Baert I, et al. Anxiety and depression in the first six months after stroke. A longitudinal multicentre study. Disabil Rehabil 2008;30(24): 1858–66.
38. Kimura M, Tateno A, Robinson RG. Treatment of poststroke generalized anxiety disorder comorbid with poststroke depression: merged analysis of nortriptyline trials. Am J Geriatr Psychiatry 2003;11(3):320–7.
39. Astrom M. Generalized anxiety disorder in stroke patients: a 3 year longitudinal study. Stroke 1996;27:270–5.
40. Kim HF, Yudofsky SC, Hales RE, et al. Neuropsychiatric aspects of seizure disorders. In: Yudofsky SC, Hales RE, editors. The american psychiatric publishing textbook of neuropsychiatry and behavioral neurosciences. Washington, DC: American Psychiatric Publishing; 2007. p. 649–76.
41. Stein M, Sherbourne C, Craske M, et al. Quality of care for primary care patients with anxiety disorders. Am J Psychiatry 2004;161:2230–7.
42. Weisberg R, Dyck I, Culpepper L, et al. Psychiatric treatment in primary care patients with anxiety disorders. Am J Psychiatry 2007;164:276–82.
43. Ravindran LM, Stein MB. Anxiety disorders: somatic treatment. In: Sadock BJ, Sadock VA, Ruiz P, editors. Kaplan and sadock's comprehensive textbook of psychiatry. 9th edition. Philadelphia: Lippincott Williams and Wilkins; 2009. p. 1906–14.
44. Huppert JD, Cahill SP, Foa EB. Anxiety disorders: cognitive-behavioral therapy. In: Sadock BJ, Sadock VA, Ruiz P, editors. Kaplan and sadock's comprehensive textbook of psychiatry. 9th edition. Philadelphia: Lippincott Williams and Wilkins; 2009. p. 1915–26.
45. Nina P, Koran L, Kiev A. High-dose sertraline strategy for nonresponders to acute treatment for obsessive-compulsive disorder. J Clin Psychiatry 2006;67:15–22.
46. Mago R, Gomez JP, Gupta N, et al. Anxiety in medically ill patients. Curr Psychiatry Rep 2006;8:228–33.
47. Stein M, Goin M, Pollack M, et al. Practice guidelines for the treatment of patients with panic disorder. Am J Psychiatry 2009;166:1–67.
48. Rosenthal L, Kim V, Kim D. Weaning from prolonged mechanical ventilation using an antipsychotic agent in a patient with acute stress disorder. Crit Care Med 2007;35:2417–9.
49. Bell C, Eth S, Friedman M, et al. Practice guideline for the treatment of patients with acute stress disorder and posttraumatic stress disorder. Am J Psychiatry 2004;161:1–31.
50. Davidson JR. Pharmacologic treatment of acute and chronic stress following trauma. J Clin Psychiatry 2006;67(2):34–9.
51. Stanley M, Wilson N, Novy D, et al. Cognitive behavior therapy for generalized anxiety disorder among older adults in primary care. JAMA 2009;301(14):1460–7.
52. Koran L, Hanna G, Hollander E, et al. Practice guideline for the treatment of patients with obsessive-compulsive disorder. Am J Psychiatry 2007;164:7–53.
53. Ludwig D, Kabat-Zinn J. Mindfulness in medicine. JAMA 2008;2000:1350–3.
54. Katon W, Roy-Byrne P, Cowley D. Cost-effectiveness and cost offset of a collaborative care intervention for primary care patient with panic disorder. Arch Gen Psychiatry 2002;12:1098–104.
55. Hollander E, Simeon D. Anxiety disorders. In: Hales RE, Yudofsky SC, editors. Textbook of clinical psychiatry. 4th edition. Washington, DC: APPI Press; 2003. p. 543–630.

An Approach to the Psychopharmacologic Care of Patients: Antidepressants, Antipsychotics, Anxiolytics, Mood Stabilizers, and Natural Remedies

Jeff C. Huffman, MD[a,b,]*, Jonathan E. Alpert, MD, PhD[a,b,c]

KEYWORDS

- Psychopharmacology • Antidepressants • Anxiolytics
- Mood stabilizers • Antipsychotics • Natural remedies

Dr Huffman has received research funding from the American Heart Association. Dr Alpert has also received research funding from the National Institute of Mental Health, National Alliance for Research on Schizophrenia and Depression (NARSAD), Abbott Laboratories, Alkermes, Lichtwer Pharma GmbH, Lorex Pharmaceuticals; Aspect Medical Systems, Astra-Zeneca, Bristol-Myers Squibb Company, Cephalon, Cyberonics, Eli Lilly & Company, Forest Pharmaceuticals Inc., GlaxoSmithKline, J & J Pharmaceuticals, Novartis, Organon Inc., PamLab, LLC, Pfizer Inc., Pharmavite, Roche, Sanofi/Synthelabo, Solvay Pharmaceuticals, Inc., and Wyeth-Ayerst Laboratories; has participated on advisory boards for or provided consultancy to Eli Lilly & Company, Pamlab LLC, and Pharmavite LLC; and has received speakers' honoraria from Eli Lilly & Company, Xian-Janssen, Organon, Belvoir Media Group, and Informa Healthcare Publisher. Drs Huffman and Alpert have received honoraria from Reed Medical Education for activities performed for the MGH Psychiatry Academy.

[a] Harvard Medical School, 260 Longwood Avenue, Boston, MA 20115, USA
[b] Department of Psychiatry, Massachusetts General Hospital, 15 Parkman Street, Boston, MA 02114, USA
[c] Depression Clinical and Research Program, Massachusetts General Hospital, 50 Staniford Street, Boston, MA 02114, USA
* Corresponding author. Department of Psychiatry, Massachusetts General Hospital, 55 Fruit Street/Blake 11, Boston, MA 02114.
E-mail address: Jhuffman@partners.org

Med Clin N Am 94 (2010) 1141–1160
doi:10.1016/j.mcna.2010.08.009
0025-7125/10/$ – see front matter © 2010 Elsevier Inc. All rights reserved.

The number of safe and effective medication treatments for psychiatric illness has expanded substantially over the past 10 to 15 years. Knowing when and how to prescribe psychotropics—and knowing which medication to prescribe—can be challenging, but with knowledge of some basic principles, this task can be performed adeptly by physicians of all specialties. In this article, the authors discuss basic principles of psychopharmacology and outline an approach to using several commonly prescribed classes of medications.

PRINCIPLES OF PSYCHOPHARMACOLOGY
Deciding to Initiate Treatment

Optimal pharmacologic treatment depends on a good working diagnosis. The use of an antidepressant alone for a college student who presents with depressed mood may be appropriate if the diagnosis is of a major depressive episode, is likely to be insufficient if the student is struggling with alcohol dependence or demoralized because of problems arising from an unaddressed learning disability, and is seriously inadequate (and possibly harmful) if the diagnosis is bipolar disorder or psychotic depression. In acute situations, it may not possible to defer pharmacotherapy until a diagnosis is fully clarified. In such situations, it is particularly important to document the differential diagnosis and the rationale for selecting a particular treatment and to specify the information needed to achieve greater diagnostic certainty, such as laboratory test results or information from collateral sources. In most circumstances, optimal care of patients with chronic or complex psychiatric syndromes involves consideration of nonmedication treatments in addition to, and sometimes instead of, pharmacologic approaches. These range from an increasingly wide array of evidence-based psychosocial treatments (eg, cognitive-behavior therapy [CBT]), lifestyle interventions (eg, improved sleep hygiene), and somatic treatments, such as electroconvulsive therapy (ECT).

Identifying Goals

Beyond clarifying the diagnosis, it is important to identify key target symptoms and goals of treatment. If treating depression, for example, the clinician should identify the symptoms that cause the most distress and that impair function, such as anhedonia, suicidal feelings, or neurovegetative symptoms (eg, fatigue, impaired concentration, or insomnia). The clinician should also elicit examples of how the symptoms are impacting quality of life and function so that the patient and clinician can serially assess the impact of treatment on these important domains.

Selecting a Treatment

Once a decision is made to use a pharmacologic approach, a specific treatment should be chosen. In many cases (eg, with antidepressants), there are multiple agents with essentially equivalent efficacy and safety. Research efforts are underway, particularly in genetics, neurophysiology, and brain imaging, to identify clinically valid and reliable predictors of response that may guide medication selection in the future. However, clinically useful biologic predictors are still lacking. An individual agent is usually chosen based on prior treatment responses, anticipated side effects, ease of dosing/monitoring, drug-drug interactions, comorbid conditions (eg, neuropathic pain, obesity) that could be affected positively or adversely, and cost. When initiating treatment, it is important to discuss certain aspects with the patient: the indication for treatment, the time when benefits are anticipated, the potential side effects/risks and their expected time course and reversibility, the laboratory monitoring required where relevant, the likely duration of treatment, the importance of regularly taking medication (whether symptoms are reduced or not), and the existence of back-up possibilities if treatment does not work (eg, other medications, psychotherapies, and nonpharmacologic somatic treatments, such as ECT). The understanding and beliefs of patients and those close to them about psychotropic medications and the illness being treated often have a major impact on treatment adherence. Time taken at the outset to explain the rationale for treatment and to address questions represents time well spent.

Monitoring the Effects of Treatment

Follow-up visits should feature efficient, systematic inquiry about key target symptoms/domains identified as relevant to the goals of treatment, safety (danger to self or others), side effects and overall tolerability of treatment, medication adherence, as well as any salient changes to general health status, psychosocial status, and use of prescription medication and over-the-counter (OTC) medications and supplements. Specific questions about common side effects (eg, sexual dysfunction or nausea) generally yield more useful information than open-ended inquiries. Likewise, nonjudgmental questions about impediments to adherence allow for more candid discussion than questions that tend to assume adherence (eg, "You're taking the medicine 3 times a day as we discussed, right?"). To determine the efficacy of a course of treatment, it is essential to aim for adequate trials in terms of duration and dose. Steady dose titration as tolerated, ongoing encouragement of adherence, and willingness to discuss and address side effects are often key components to achieve this goal.

Discontinuing Treatment

When discussing discontinuation of treatment with a patient, the risks of stopping medication must be discussed, especially the risk of relapse once off the medication and the plan for monitoring for that risk. The method of discontinuation must also be carefully considered, because some psychotropic medications are associated with withdrawal or "discontinuation emergent" symptoms on sudden cessation, and even without a medication-specific withdrawal syndrome, relapse rates may be higher if treatment is abruptly stopped.[1-3] These associated risks of discontinuing treatment must be weighed against the benefits (eg, reducing side-effect burden, potential drug interactions, cost, inconvenience).

Approach to Treatment Failure

Several factors may play a role in treatment failure.

The patient's *diagnosis* may be incorrect, or there may be critical comorbid conditions (eg, substance use disorders) that may prevent resolution of symptoms (or efficacy of medication). The *dose* of the medication may be suboptimal because of inadequate dosing, problems with adherence, or pharmacokinetic issues (eg, concurrent use of metabolic inducers, such as carbamazepine). *Drugs*, both prescribed and illicit, can affect ongoing symptoms (eg, effects of steroids, such as prednisone, on mood) or influence drug levels (eg, effects of thiazide diuretics or high-dose nonsteroidal anti-inflammatory agents [NSAIDs] on lithium levels). Finally, *disruptions*—psychosocial stressors—may also be potential impediments to treatment and should be met with aggressive efforts to ensure the adequacy of pharmacologic treatment and with equally determined efforts to develop a plan for addressing the environmental factors that seem to be compromising a patient's recovery.

ANTIDEPRESSANTS

There are several commonly used classes of antidepressants. These include the selective serotonin reuptake inhibitors (SSRIs), the serotonin and norepinephrine reuptake inhibitors (SNRIs), and the atypical antidepressants (eg, bupropion and mirtazapine); **Table 1** summarizes indications, dosing, and side effects of these treatments. Older classes of antidepressants (tricyclic antidepressants [TCAs] and monoamine oxidase inhibitors [MAOIs]) are still used occasionally. Overall, most of the evidence suggests that these agents are roughly equivalent in the treatment of depression,[4–6] and therefore, agent selection is often based on comorbid conditions, side-effect profiles, treatment history, and cost.

SSRIs

The SSRIs are the most commonly prescribed antidepressants. All SSRIs share similar pharmacologic actions, including minimal anticholinergic, antihistaminic, and α_1-adrenergic blocking effects, and potent presynaptic inhibition of serotonin reuptake. They are generally well-tolerated and are not as dangerous in overdose as are the older agents, and many are available generically. The starting dose can serve as an initial target dose, and SSRIs are generally taken once daily. Another advantage is that they are effective for major depression, dysthymia, and nearly every anxiety disorder, including generalized anxiety disorder (GAD), post-traumatic stress disorder (PTSD), obsessive-compulsive disorder (OCD), and panic disorder (PD). Only minor differences exist among the specific agents: citalopram, escitalopram, and sertraline have the lowest risk of drug-drug interactions; whereas paroxetine is more often sedating and has more anticholinergic effects; paroxetine and fluoxetine are potent inhibitors of cytochrome P450 2D6, requiring caution when coprescribing with certain substrates (eg, antiarrhythmics, lipophilic β-blockers, and TCAs); and fluvoxamine inhibits cytochrome P450 1A2 and 3A4, requiring caution when coprescribing with a range of medications (including theophylline, cyclosporine, midazolam, calcium channel-blockers, and pimozide). When stopped abruptly, SSRIs can be associated with a discontinuation syndrome, with associated influenza-like symptoms (dizziness, nausea, headache), parasthesias, and sleep disturbance.[7] The syndrome is uncomfortable but not dangerous and is most common with SSRIs having the shortest half-life (paroxetine and fluvoxamine); it is exceedingly rare with fluoxetine, which has a long-acting metabolite. Finally, use of SSRIs in pregnant women must be carefully considered; these agents may be associated with some neurobehavioral disturbances in the postpartum period (and paroxetine with persistent pulmonary hypertension of the newborn),[8] but untreated depression—and discontinuation of effective treatment—are also associated with poor maternal and neonatal outcomes.[9]

SNRIs

Blocking the reuptake of serotonin and norepinephrine, the two most commonly used SNRIs, venlafaxine and duloxetine, have been joined by desvenlafaxine, a metabolite of venlafaxine more recently approved for treatment of major depressive disorder. Like the SSRIs, these agents are generally well-tolerated and safer than older agents in overdose; venlafaxine is available generically. SNRIs are effective for depression and some anxiety disorders (eg, venlafaxine in GAD), although they have been much less well-studied than SSRIs for anxiety disorders. Venlafaxine and probably desvenlafaxine and duloxetine are associated with dose-dependent increases in blood pressure[10,11]; all three associated with a discontinuation syndrome. Duloxetine, like paroxetine and fluoxetine, is an inhibitor of cytochrome P450 2D6. SNRIs are

Table 1
Antidepressants

Agent	Typical Daily Starting Dose	Target Daily Dose	Side Effects	Other Features
SSRIs				
Citalopram	20 mg	20–80 mg	Nausea, anxiety, tremor, sedation, insomnia, headache, sexual dysfunction	Few drug-drug interactions
Escitalopram	10 mg	10–40 mg	Same as previous	Few drug-drug interactions
Fluoxetine	20 mg	20–80 mg	Same as previous	Low risk of discontinuation syndrome; cytochrome P450 2D6 inhibition
Fluvoxamine	50–100 mg	50–300 mg	Same as previous; possibly higher rates of gastrointestinal side effects	Short half-life; higher risk of discontinuation syndrome; cytochrome P450 1A2 and 3A4 inhibition
Paroxetine	20 mg	20–80 mg	Same as previous; possibly higher rates of sedation; mild anticholinergic side effects	Short half-life; higher risk of discontinuation syndrome; cytochrome P450 2D6 inhibition
Sertraline	50–100 mg	50–300 mg	Same as previous; possibly higher rates of gastrointestinal side effects	Few drug-drug interactions; moderate cytochrome P450 2D6 inhibition
SNRIs				
Desvenlafaxine	50 mg	50–100 mg	Nausea, headache, dizziness, dry mouth insomnia, sedation, sexual dysfunction	Probable dose-dependent increase in blood pressure; probable association with discontinuation syndrome
Duloxetine	20–40 mg	60–120 mg	Same as previous	Associated with rare increase in liver function tests; cytochrome P450 2D6 inhibition
Venlafaxine	37.5–75 mg	150–300 mg	Same as previous	Dose-dependent increase in blood pressure can occur; high rates of discontinuation syndrome if stopped abruptly
Atypical antidepressants				
Bupropion	100–200 mg	300–450 mg	Headache, insomnia, tremor, anxiety; lower risk of sexual dysfunction than SSRIs	Increased risk of seizure at doses>450 mg/d; Cytochrome P450 2D6 inhibition
Mirtazapine	15 mg	15–45 mg	Sedation, increased appetite, weight gain, mild orthostasis	Can be associated with increases in lipids

not well-studied in pregnant patients and should be used with caution. Dual reuptake inhibitors, like the older TCAs, such as amitriptyline, but unlike the SSRIs, seem to have a role in the treatment of pain syndromes, particularly neuropathic pain, and are therefore often considered for treatment of depressed patients with comorbid pain.

Atypical Antidepressants

Mirtazapine, a serotonin-receptor blocker that also has effects on norepinephrine via blockade of α_2-adrenergic receptors, and bupropion, an agent with effects on norepinephrine and dopamine, represent important alternatives to the SSRIs and SNRIs and, for treatment-resistant depression, are sometimes used in combination with them in more complex pharmacologic regimens. Both are used primarily for the treatment of depression, evidence for their efficacy in anxiety disorders being sparse; bupropion has been found to be effective as an agent for smoking cessation and also is particularly unlikely to cause sexual dysfunction. However, bupropion, like some of the SSRIs and SNRIs, is a potent inhibitor of cytochrome P450 2D6. Mirtazapine causes significant blockade at histamine (H_1) receptors and 5-HT_2 receptors, leading to sedation and increased appetite/weight gain; this may be problematic for many patients but it can be beneficial for patients who sleep and eat poorly. Bupropion, in contrast, is not associated with sedation or weight gain but may be associated with insomnia, jitteriness, or anxiety. Both agents are relatively safe in overdose, although bupropion has also been associated with an increased risk of seizures at higher than recommended doses (single doses higher than 150 mg of the immediate-release formulation, 200 mg of the sustained-release formulation, or higher than 450 mg/d), and seizure is a risk with bupropion overdose as well as in patients at risk of seizure, such as those with a central nervous system lesion or active eating disorder. Neither agent is well-studied in pregnancy.

TCAs and MAOIs

These older agents are limited by their greater risk in overdose, potential effects on cardiac conduction/arrhythmias (TCAs), and substantial required restrictions on diet and medications (MAOIs). TCAs are also associated with orthostatic hypotension, sedation, and anticholinergic effects, and MAOIs commonly cause orthostasis as well. TCAs are still sometimes used at low doses for sleep or neuropathic pain, and an MAOI (selegeline) patch has been developed that does not require dietary restriction at the lowest available dose, although restrictions on several drug classes are still required, even at the lowest dose.

Practical approaches to treatment

For many patients, including those with anxiety disorders (in isolation or with comorbid depression), SSRIs are a natural first-line choice among antidepressants. There are, however, specific situations in which using a different class of agent may make sense (eg, patients who are trying to quit smoking or have had problems with sexual dysfunction on serotonergic agents [bupropion], patients who have very poor appetite and sleep [mirtazapine], or patients with comorbid neuropathic pain [duloxetine]). When prescribing antidepressants, the lowest usual therapeutic dose is customarily considered (eg, citalopram 20 mg), but if there is less than 20% to 30% improvement over the ensuing 2 to 4 weeks and adequate tolerability, the dose should be pushed upward. If a depressed patient has a minimal response to an adequately and aggressively dosed trial of an SSRI or is unable to tolerate the medication, switching to a second SSRI or another class of agent (eg, SNRI or bupropion) seems to be equally effective.[5] If the patient has a partial response to the maximally tolerated dose of an SSRI, rather than switching agents, many clinicians choose to continue the SSRI and add a second antidepressant, usually bupropion or mirtazapine, or consider adding a nonantidepressant with evidence for efficacy as augmentation of antidepressants. Various nonantidepressant agents have been used as augmenting agents (including lithium, triiodothyronine [T3] dopamine agonists, such as pramipexole, buspirone, the antianxiety agent, and psychostimulants, such as methylphenidate) with varying degrees of evidence. However, in recent years, the atypical antipsychotics (eg, aripiprazole, quetiapine, olanzapine) have received particularly active attention as well as Food and Drug Administration-approval for antidepressant augmentation. Nevertheless, their risks, particularly of metabolic syndrome and extrapyramidal side effects, and their costs must be considered in each case.

ANXIOLYTICS AND SLEEP AGENTS
Benzodiazepines

The most commonly used antianxiety agents are benzodiazepines (**Table 2**).They are agonists at specific γ-aminobutyric acid $(GABA)_A$ receptors and are used for various symptoms and syndromes that include free-floating anxiety, PD, insomnia, and muscle spasm. Benzodiazepines have the advantage of being rapidly effective but have several caveats associated with their use. They have been associated with increased risk of falls, development of delirium (especially in persons with pre-existing cognitive disorders), and potential for respiratory depression.[12] Furthermore, long-term use of these agents leads to physiologic dependence, and if and when discontinued, they require tapering off. Because of these disadvantages, the SSRIs and SNRIs have become the mainstay of longer-term treatment of many anxiety disorders (including PD, GAD, social anxiety, OCD, and PTSD). Because of the potential for developing dependence, benzodiazepine use for patients with prior or ongoing substance-use disorders must be considered carefully. However, when these agents are used at appropriate doses for appropriate indications (eg, PD), they are effective, and dose escalation does not typically occur.[13] Selection of a specific benzodiazepine depends on several factors. For example, diazepam and clonazepam have longer half-lives, allowing less frequent dosing and less fluctuation of blood levels; these agents are widely used for patients who need standing treatment throughout the day (eg, PD). In contrast, lorazepam and oxazepam are shorter-acting and may be more beneficial when used as-needed for insomnia or for patients with impaired hepatic metabolism. These agents have been used effectively in pregnant women, although they may be associated with low birth weight and neonatal sedation in the child.[14]

Short-Acting GABA_A Agents

The agents zolpidem, zaleplon, and eszopiclone are short-acting agents used specifically for insomnia. These sedative-hypnotics are $GABA_A$ receptor agonists but do not act on the benzodiazepine receptor per se and have shorter half-lives than most benzodiazepines. These agents are effective in the treatment of insomnia and are usually well-tolerated. Although they have less risk of physiologic dependence than benzodiazepines, at high doses, dependence and a withdrawal syndrome can occur.[15] One set of potentially adverse effects associated with these medications is related to nocturnal behaviors; a small subset of patients taking these medications engage in sleepwalking, nighttime eating, or more complex behaviors that occur during sleep; the patient is typically amnestic for these events.[16,17] This syndrome

Table 2
Anxiety and sleep agents

Agent	Typical Daily Starting Dose (and typical dose for prn use)	Typical Daily Target Dose	Speed of Onset	Duration of Effect	Potential Side Effects	Other Considerations
Benzodiazepines						
Alprazolam	0.25–1 mg	1.5–3 mg	Rapid	Short	Sedation, ataxia, confusion, respiratory depression	
Clonazepam	0.25–1 mg	1.5–3 mg	Slow	Long	Same	
Diazepam	2.5–5 mg	10–20 mg	Rapid	Long	Same	Active metabolites
Lorazepam	0.5–1 mg	2–5 mg	Moderate	Short	Same	Undergoes reduced hepatic metabolism; better choice in patients with hepatic insufficiency
Oxazepam	15 mg	15–30 mg	Moderate	Short	Same	Undergoes reduced hepatic metabolism
GABA$_A$ sleep agents						
Eszopiclone	2 mg	2–3 mg	Rapid	Short	Sedation, dizziness, headache, unpleasant taste	Potential risk of nocturnal eating behavior and somnambulism.
Zaleplon	5–10 mg	10 mg	Rapid	Very Short	Sedation, dizziness, headache	Same previous
Zolpidem	5 mg	5–10 mg	Rapid	Short	Sedation, dizziness, headache	Most associated with amnestic nocturnal eating and somnambulism
Other agents						
Buspirone	10–20 mg	30–45 mg	Slow	Long	Headache, dizziness	Used for GAD
Ramelteon	8 mg	8–16 mg	Rapid	Short	Sedation	Sleep agent
Trazodone	25–50 mg	25–100 mg	Moderate	Moderate	Sedation, headache, orthostasis	Used for sleep; Risk of priapism in men (1/6000)

has most frequently been observed with the use of zolpidem. Although rare, it is important to warn patients of these potential effects.

Other Sleep and Anxiety Agents

Trazodone is an antagonist at serotonin and α_{-1} receptors. It was initially marketed as an antidepressant but is now more frequently used to treat insomnia. It is generally effective and well-tolerated, although it can cause daytime sedation, orthostatic hypotension, and, very rarely, priapism in men. Ramelteon is a sleep agent with a different mechanism—it is a melatonin-receptor agonist, and it may be helpful with insomnia or shifted sleep-wake cycles. Overall, ramelteon is quite well-tolerated but, clinically, tends to be less effective in actively inducing sleep than other agents.[18] Finally, buspirone is an agent that was developed for the treatment of GAD; it has the advantage of being very well-tolerated and having no risk of physiologic dependence. However, although it has been used for GAD and as an adjunct to antidepressant treatment of depression, some clinicians find that it has limited effectiveness, particularly for patients who have been treated previously with benzodiazepines.

Practical approach to treatment

With respect to the pharmacologic treatment of anxiety, assessing the nature of the anxiety before embarking on treatment is critical. Specifically, does the patient have a formal anxiety disorder (eg, GAD or PD) or simply periods of anxiety? Brief situational anxiety or certain phobias (eg, flying) can be reasonably well treated with a brief course of benzodiazepines, often at low doses, although behavioral approaches are highly effective and should be considered for patients with recurrent difficulty with situational anxiety or simple phobias. Panic disorder is often rapidly responsive to moderate-to-high–dose benzodiazepines, such as clonazepam (which may be used on a standing basis), although is also treated over the longer-term with SSRIs because of the potential risks associated with chronic benzodiazepine use. On the other hand, other anxiety disorders (eg, OCD, GAD, PTSD) are often better treated primarily with SSRIs (or SNRIs), sometimes with benzodiazepines for augmentation. With insomnia treatment, it is likewise helpful to determine if the insomnia occurs in the context of another psychiatric illness (eg, depression) or a medical disorder (eg, restless legs syndrome or obstructive sleep apnea) to determine if targeted treatment of the underlying illness is needed. Polysomnography should be considered for persistent sleep disturbance of unclear cause. If insomnia is the primary problem and sleep hygiene techniques do not help, first-line options include the use of short-acting GABA agents, like zolpidem (which have lesser impact on rapid eye movement (REM) sleep than other agents and do not tend to cause oversedation) or trazodone (which may impact REM sleep more and is longer-acting but is not associated with nighttime behaviors).[19] Although short-term treatment of insomnia is ideal, some patients, particularly those with comorbid psychiatric and medical conditions (eg, chronic pain) that may cause persistent challenges to sleep, seem to require maintenance standing sleep medication using the lowest effective dose of sedative-hypnotic and ongoing monitoring to reassess risks and benefits.

MOOD STABILIZERS
Lithium

Among the mood stabilizers—agents used to prevent or treat manic or depressive episodes among patients with bipolar disorder—lithium has been used the longest and, in some ways, remains the gold standard of this class, particularly for *classic* bipolar disorder characterized by distinct episodes of full mania and depression

(**Table 3**). The mechanism by which lithium and the other mood stabilizers work remains unclear and may be the result of effects on neurotransmitters or other, more upstream effects (eg, on gene expression). Lithium can be used to treat the manic and depressive phases of illness, and as a maintenance agent, it has been shown to reduce the risk of suicide.[20] However, initiation and continuation of lithium must be considered and monitored carefully, given that this agent is also associated with multiple side effects, has a narrow therapeutic index, and is involved in multiple clinically significant drug-drug interactions. In addition to more common side effects (eg, tremor, weight gain, cognitive dulling, and polydipsia/polyuria), lithium is also associated with the development of hypothyroidism and with the gradual development of renal insufficiency/failure. At levels higher than the therapeutic range (generally considered to be 0.6–1 mEq/L), toxicity can begin, with the onset of symptoms typically around 1.5 mEq/L and more serious symptoms, including stupor, dysarthria, severe tremor, ataxia, and delirium, at higher levels. Given these risks, it is important to follow lithium levels (especially during initiation and dose changes) and to systematically monitor renal function every 3 to 6 months. Also, several commonly prescribed medications, including prescription-strength NSAIDs, angiotensin-converting enzyme inhibitors, and thiazide diuretics, can increase lithium levels and lead to toxicity, whereas aminophylline and theophylline may cause lithium levels to decrease. Use of lithium during pregnancy is associated with an elevated risk of Ebstein anomaly[21]; however, it otherwise does not appear to be associated with major malformations and is generally considered to be the treatment of choice among pregnant women with bipolar disorder, although levels need to be monitored closely because of fluid/volume shifts during the course of pregnancy.[22]

Anticonvulsant Mood Stabilizers

Valproic acid is the anticonvulsant for which there is the most evidence of efficacy in bipolar disorder, especially for the treatment of acute manic episodes and as maintenance treatment to reduce risk of relapse into mania or depression. It is sometimes used more generally for the treatment of impulsivity and aggression. Valproic acid can be titrated much more aggressively than lithium for manic patients, has a much wider therapeutic index, and is less dangerous in toxicity/overdose. However, it still can have side effects—sedation, weight gain, gastrointestinal (GI) upset, and diarrhea are among the most common—and can less commonly be associated with elevations in liver function tests and with platelet dysfunction. Hyperammonemia or pancreatitis may present emergently though rarely on valproic acid use. With regard to drug-drug interactions, it can slow the metabolism of aspirin, warfarin, lamotrigine, and some benzodiazepines (eg, diazepam), increasing levels of those medications. Valproic acid has been strongly associated with neural tube defects and generally should be avoided in pregnant women.

Lamotrigine is effective in the treatment of bipolar depression and in preventing recurrent mood episodes, especially depression. It is well-tolerated, does not have significant associated weight gain, sedation, or GI side effects, and does not require monitoring with laboratory tests. However, rapid titration of lamotrigine is associated with dangerous dermatologic conditions, including Stevens-Johnson syndrome, and therefore, the dose must be slowly increased over the course of many weeks; patients should be told to contact their physician with any rash associated with lamotrigine use. Concomitant use of valproic acid, which is common in the management of patients with refractory bipolar states, requires a slower rate of lamotrigine titration to avoid this risk. Based on limited available information, use of lamotrigine in pregnant women seems to be associated with elevated rates of oral clefts.[23]

Table 3
Lithium and selected anticonvulsant mood stabilizers

Agent	Typical Daily Starting Dose	Typical Daily Target Dose	Therapeutic Level	Potential Side Effects	Selected Drug-Drug Interactions	Monitoring
Lithium	300–600 mg	900–1800 mg	0.6–1.0 mEq/L (trough)	Tremor, GI upset, polydipsia, polyuria, weight gain, sedation cognitive slowing, acne, edema, hypothyroidism, hypercalcemia, renal failure	Thiazide diuretics, high-dose NSAIDs, ACE inhibitors, and A-II blockers increase lithium levels Aminophylline, theophylline, loop diuretics, and carbonic anhydrase inhibitors may decrease lithium levels	*During initiation:* baseline BUN/creatinine, TSH, follow lithium levels with dose titration *Maintenance:* Serum creatinine every 3–6 months; TSH annually With change in clinical state, check lithium level and TSH (if patient depressed)
Valproic acid	250–500 mg	1000–2000 mg	50–100 + mcg/mL (trough)	GI upset, tremor, sedation, dizziness, weight gain, alopecia, elevated ammonia, elevated LFTs, platelet dysfunction, pancreatitis	Depakote increases levels of: lamotrigine, carbamazepine, aspirin, warfarin, diazepam, clonazepam Valproic acid levels decreased by: phenytoin, carbamazepine, topiramate	*During initiation:* baseline LFTs and CBC; follow levels with dose titration *Maintenance:* LFTs/CBC every 3–6 months With change in clinical state, check level
Lamotrigine	25 mg	100–400 mg	Not routinely used	Headache, nausea, rash, serious dermatologic syndrome (eg, Stevens-Johnson syndrome)	Lamotrigine levels increased by valproic acid (use half daily dose of lamotrigine when coadministered) and decreased by carbamazepine	None

Abbreviations: ACE, angiotensin-converting enzyme; A-II, angiotensin-II; BUN, blood urea nitrogen; CBC, complete blood count; GI, gastrointestinal; LFTs, liver function tests; TSH, thyrotropin.

Carbamazepine and the related compound oxcarbazepine have also been used in the treatment of patients with bipolar disorder; they (particularly oxcarbazepine) may be less effective than valproic acid for manic symptoms and less effective than lamotrigine for depression. One advantage of these agents is that they are not—in contrast to most other mood stabilizers—associated with significant weight gain. Both agents are associated with hyponatremia; carbamazepine, and, to a lesser degree, oxcarbazepine, can induce the metabolism of medications, especially those metabolized by the 3A4 isoenzyme of the cytochrome P450 system (eg, immunosuppressants, protease inhibitors, and oral contraceptives [OCPs]). Indeed, both agents can induce the metabolism of OCPs, and patients should be told to use another form of contraception, especially given the risk of neural tube defects associated with carbamazepine and possibly oxcarbazepine. Carbamazepine has also been associated with aplastic anemia and dermatologic side effects, including development of Stevens-Johnson syndrome. Finally, other anticonvulsants (eg, topiramate, gabapentin) seem to be less effective as mood stabilizers than those listed earlier, and their role in bipolar disorder is generally reserved for targeting other co-occurring conditions for which they may be effective.

Practical approach to the use of mood stabilizers

In addition to lithium and the anticonvulsants discussed earlier, several atypical antipsychotics have been shown to be effective in the management of mood episodes in bipolar disorder, even in the absence of psychotic symptoms. Although these agents have a much less narrow therapeutic index than lithium or carbamazepine and do not require therapeutic-level monitoring, they do entail risk of metabolic syndrome, which requires ongoing monitoring, and there is a risk of extrapyramidal symptoms (EPSs). Overall, when selecting a specific pharmacologic agent to treat a patient with bipolar disorder, it is often helpful to consider the patient's current clinical state. For acute *mania*, valproic acid and atypical antipsychotics can be titrated upward most rapidly and are often considered to be first-line agents; lithium can also be used, but it is typically paired with a second agent that can be used to quell symptoms while lithium is being more gradually titrated upward. For patients with acute *bipolar depression*, lithium, lamotrigine, and quetiapine, the atypical antipsychotic, are often considered to be first-line agents. Finally, for patients who are currently stable but who require maintenance treatment of bipolar disorder, lithium is the treatment of choice for those who can safely take this medication; valproic acid and several atypical antipsychotics (eg, olanzapine or aripiprazole) are also reasonable options. Given the significant short- and long-term side effects that can be associated with all these medications and the need for laboratory monitoring with many of them, the patient and clinician should carefully consider the risks, benefits, and potential side effects of the reasonable available options and come to a collaborative decision. Although antidepressants are not infrequently used for bipolar depression, their efficacy in bipolar disorder remains uncertain, and their use is thought to increase the risk of mania, rapid cycling, or mixed manic/depressive states for some patients. Antidepressants should generally be used sparingly in the treatment of patients with bipolar disorder and only in the setting of adequate mood stabilization with other agents.

ANTIPSYCHOTICS
Typical Antipsychotics

This older class of antipsychotic agents, which include haloperidol, fluphenazine, and perphenazine, work by blocking dopamine D_2 receptors (**Table 4**). Currently, these medications are used much less frequently than the newer atypical antipsychotics.

Table 4
Antipsychotic medications

Agent	Initial Daily Dose (mg)	Target Daily Dose^c (mg)	Sedation	Orthostasis	Ach	EPS	TD	Weight Gain	Metabolic Effects	Hyper PRL
Perphenazine	4–16	16–64	++	++	++	++	++	++	+	++
Fluphenazine	2.5–5	5–15	+	0	0	++++	++	+	+	++
Haloperidol	2.5–5	5–15	+	0	0	++++	++	+	+	++
Risperidone	1–2	3–6	+	+++	0	+++	+	++	++	+++
Paliperidone	6	6–12	+	++	0	+++	?	++	++	+++
Iloperidone^b	2	12–24	+	+++	0	++	?	+	+	++
Ziprasidone	40–80	120–240	0	+	0	++	?	0	0	0
Asenapine^b	5–10	10–20	++	+	0	+/++	?	+	+	+
Olanzapine	5–10	10–30	++	0	+/++	+/++	+	++++	++++	+
Aripiprazole	5–15	15–30	0/+	0	0	++^a	?	0	0	0
Quetiapine	25–50	300–800	+++	++	0	0	0?	++	++	0
Clozapine	25	200–450	++++	++++	+++	0	0?	++++	++++	0

Abbreviations: Ach, anticholinergic; EPS, extrapyramidal symptoms; PRL, prolactin; TD, tardive dyskinesia.
^a When used for schizophrenia spectrum disorders; doses may differ for other indications.
^b New agent; limited clinical data regarding side effects is available.
^c Akathisia only.

The typical antipsychotics are used primarily for the treatment of schizophrenia spectrum disorders; however, they can be used to treat patients with psychotic symptoms associated with other syndromes, including psychotic depression (in combination with an antidepressant), mania with psychotic features, and delirium. They have fallen somewhat out of favor because of side effects that can include EPSs (dystonia, parkinsonism, and akathisia) and tardive dyskinesia (TD; a long-term, relatively irreversible side effect causing involuntary motor movements) and, rarely, neuroleptic malignant syndrome. However, these medications are very effective in the treatment of psychosis, and large studies have found that they may be as effective as the atypical antipsychotics in the treatment of schizophrenia.[24] Furthermore, they can usually be dosed once daily, and particularly the higher-potency agents (eg, haloperidol) seem to have lesser metabolic side effects than some of the atypical antipsychotics. There is more evidence for their relative safety in pregnancy than the atypical antipsychotics.[22] Particularly at high doses, there is a risk of arrhythmia accompanying use of the low-potency agents (eg, chlorpromazine, thioridazine) and some of the other agents (eg, pimozide and intravenous haloperidol or droperidol).

Atypical Antipsychotics

This class of antipsychotics is differentiated from the typical ones by their blockade of serotonin 5-HT_{2A} receptors and by lack of a linear relationship between clinical potency and D_2-receptor blockade; some agents (eg, risperidone) have substantial effects on D_2 receptors, whereas others (eg, quetiapine) having almost none, although acting on other dopamine receptors. The atypical antipsychotic aripiprazole, rather than blocking dopamine receptors, is a partial dopamine receptor agonist. Overall, atypical antipsychotics are effective for all conditions treated by typical antipsychotics, and many seem to be effective in patients with bipolar disorder for acute mania and as maintenance mood stabilizers. These agents vary in their side effects but, overall, have a lower risk of TD compared with the typical antipsychotics and, in general, are rather well-tolerated. Metabolic side effects, however, have become a major concern with some of these agents, with associations between the agents and the development of metabolic syndrome (including weight gain, hyperlipidemia, and development of diabetes). Metabolic side effects seem to be greatest with clozapine and olanzapine, intermediate with risperidone/paliperidone and quetiapine, and relatively minimal with ziprasidone and aripiprazole.[25] Given these concerns, patients taking atypical antipsychotics should have regular monitoring of weight, blood pressure, lipids, and blood glucose.[26] Clozapine, because of its potential to cause agranulocytosis in up to 1% of patients, has restrictive prescribing and monitoring requirements, such that patients must have their white blood cell count measured weekly for the first 5 months and every other week for the remainder of treatment. These agents are not yet well-studied in pregnancy, and the older typical agents are generally used to treat and prevent psychotic symptoms in pregnancy.

Two antipsychotics have recently been introduced in the United States. Iloperidone blocks serotonin 5-HT_{2A} receptors and, to a lesser degree, D_2 receptors; pharmacologically, it seems somewhat similar to risperidone, although it seems to be associated with fewer EPSs; orthostasis with initial use requires slow titration of iloperidone to the target dose. Asenapine works via blockade of multiple serotonin and dopamine receptors; it seems to have potentially lower risk of weight gain than most atypical antipsychotics, although associated with akathisia and other EPSs. The relative benefits of these agents compared with other atypical antipsychotics are yet to be determined.

Practical approach to the use of antipsychotics

In general, most antipsychotics are equally effective in the treatment of psychotic disorders, and therefore, decision-making about specific medications revolves around side effects, long-term effects, cost, and other practical issues. Also, a limited subset of antipsychotics are available for intravenous administration, particularly helpful in intensive care unit settings; others are available in long-acting injectable depot form for longer-term use as noted in later discussion. When possible, the pros and cons of several agents should be discussed with patients and their families. When dosing with these agents, it is important to maintain a balance: one must allow time for these medications to have an effect (especially when dealing with long-held delusional beliefs and/or chronic schizophrenia spectral illness, which can take quite some time to respond); it is also important to ensure that a systematic up-titration of dose is undertaken if symptoms are not fully responding to the current dose. The frequency and rate of dose increase depends on the severity and acuity of psychotic symptoms—possibly every few days. more often for a patient with acute psychotic symptoms necessitating psychiatric admission, or monthly for patients with chronic symptoms that do not profoundly impact function.

Long-acting injectable forms of antipsychotics (eg, long-acting haloperidol, fluphenazine, risperidone, paliperidone, and olanzapine) should be considered fairly early in the course of treatment to avoid unnecessary morbidity and, ideally, to improve the course of illness for patients experiencing serious relapses related to recurrent noncompliance with medication; this is a not infrequent challenge, often linked to poor insight inherent in psychotic illness. For patients who do not respond to adequate trials of multiple antipsychotics, clozapine does, in fact, seem to be more effective than the other agents for refractory psychotic disorders and some severe mood disorders, and it should be considered in such patients; however, its multiple serious side effects, risks of seizure and agranulocytosis, and need for ongoing hematological monitoring generally relegate it to being used only for these refractory cases.

NATURAL REMEDIES

Several preparations of natural remedies, available OTC as dietary health supplements without formal illness indication, have been formally studied to assess their impact on psychiatric conditions (**Table 5**). In many cases, the studies have not found these treatments to be greatly effective, but these agents may help some patients with mood symptoms, anxiety, and insomnia, particularly those who are reluctant to take prescription medications, have not responded to or tolerated adequate trials of better-established agents previously, or wish to cautiously augment their regimen with these other agents. Given their popularity and widespread use among patients with psychiatric conditions, it is crucial for clinicians to ask patients whether they are taking OTC supplements because of their potential interactions with prescribed medications.

Agents Used for Depression

Natural agents used for depression include S-adenosylmethionine (SAMe), Omega-3 fatty acids, and St John's wort. SAMe is involved in the methylation of neurotransmitters, nucleic acids, proteins, and phospholipids; its role in the production of serotonin, norepinephrine, and dopamine may best explain SAMe's putative antidepressant properties.[27] Several meta-analyses have found SAMe to be more effective than placebo in the treatment of unipolar depression, although at generally high doses.[28] SAMe is generally well-tolerated; however, serotonin syndrome (SS), characterized

Table 5
Selected natural remedies used to treat psychiatric symptoms

Agent	Used to Treat	Target Dose	Side Effects	Potential Drug-Drug Interactions
SAMe	Depression	800–1600 mg/d	Mild anxiety, agitation, insomnia, dry mouth, GI disturbance	Possible SS when combined with antidepressants or other serotonergic drugs
St John's wort (Hypericum perforatum)	Depression	900–1800 mg/d	Dry mouth, dizziness, GI disturbance, phototoxicity	Reduced levels of certain critical drugs, such as immunosuppressants, warfarin, antiretrovirals, and digoxin. Also possible SS with serotonergic drugs
Omega-3 fatty acids (primarily EPA and DHA)	Depression	1000–2000 mg/d (EPA and/or DHA)	GI disturbance, fishy taste	
Kava (Piper methysticum)	Anxiety (and insomnia)	60–120 mg/d	GI disturbance, headache, dizziness, ataxia, oral hypoesthesia rash, potential for hepatotoxicity	Oversedation possible with other sedating medications, especially those that also have effects at GABA receptors (eg, benzodiazepines)
Melatonin	Insomnia	0.25–0.3 mg/d	Sedation, headache, nausea, dizziness, irritability	
Ginkgo biloba	Cognitive disturbance	120–240 mg/d	Mild GI disturbance, headache, irritability, dizziness, increased risk of bleeding	Potentially elevated risk of bleeding when coadministered with anticoagulant or antiplatelet agents

Abbreviations: DHA, docosahexaenoic acid; EPA, eicosapentaenoic acid; SAMe, S-adenosylmethionine; SS, serotonin syndrome.

by confusion, fever, myoclonus, and hyperreflexia, may be a risk when SAMe is combined with highly serotonergic agents. Nevertheless, several small trials have been undertaken in which SAMe has been used to safely augment SSRIs and SNRIs. Omega-3 fatty acids, which may work by affecting neurotransmitter signaling, regulating calcium channels, lowering plasma norepinephrine, or inhibiting secretion of inflammatory cytokines, have been studied for patients with both unipolar and bipolar depression, with generally positive but somewhat mixed results. At this stage, it is generally thought that the best evidence points to use of these agents to augment standard treatments rather than to be used as montotherapy.[29] St John's wort may work by the inhibition of cytokines, a decrease in serotonin receptor density, a decrease in reuptake of neurotransmitters, and weak MAOI activity.[27] Overall, St John's wort seems to be effective for milder forms of depression but may be less effective than standard agents in the treatment of more serious depression.[27,30] Initial concerns about the risk of SS when combined with serotonergic agents have only been weakly borne out. However, case reports and clinical trials indicate that some critical medications may be rendered less effective in some patients concurrently taking St John's wort. These medications include immunosuppressants (eg, cyclosporine and tacrolimus), warfarin, antiretrovirals, digoxin, and oral contraceptives.

Agents used for Anxiety, Sleep, and Memory

Kava is a natural remedy for anxiety; its mechanism may be attributable to kavapyrones, which are central muscle relaxants that are thought to be involved in blockade of voltage-gated sodium ion channels, enhanced binding to $GABA_A$ receptors, diminished excitatory neurotransmitter release, and reduced reuptake of norepinephrine. Kava's use has been much reduced over the last several years because of concerns that it may lead to hepatotoxicity.[31] Melatonin is a hormone made in the pineal gland that has been shown to help travelers avoid jet lag and to decrease sleep latency for those suffering from insomnia; it may also help night-shift workers maintain regular sleep-wake cycles. Melatonin is derived from serotonin and is thought to play a role in the organization of circadian rhythms. Finally, *Ginkgo biloba* is a natural remedy made from the seed of the Ginkgo tree that has been used to address cognitive impairment and enhance memory; it may work via neuronal stimulation/protection and scavenging of free radicals. Although some studies have found benefit for these agents in modestly improving memory in demented and nondemented patients, overall, the evidence for such benefit remains mixed.[32] Ginkgo has been associated with an increased risk of bleeding; therefore, it should be used with caution in patients at risk of bleeding or those taking anticoagulant medications.

Practical approach to natural remedies

The most important thing regarding natural remedies is for clinicians to regularly ask patients about their use and to be aware of their potential interactions with prescribed medications, psychiatric and nonpsychiatric. Also, as federal regulation of dietary health supplements differs markedly from that of prescription medications, it is helpful for patients to know that marked differences in bioavailability may exist across different brands and formulations of a given product. Nevertheless, inherent in the doctor-patient relationship is a commitment to negotiating treatment decisions with the patient in the context of available evidence about risks and benefits. In the setting of patient interest in discussing OTC remedies and other possible complementary and integrative approaches, the willingness of a clinician to address their use thoughtfully, albeit cautiously, and with acknowledgment of limited data and expertise, may reinforce a patient's trust and treatment adherence.

SUMMARY

A growing range of safe and effective pharmacologic treatments allows for increasingly targeted and resourceful care of patients with psychiatric conditions. In many cases, these treatments will be delivered alongside other care, including psychotherapies and lifestyle interventions as well as other medical care; this requires coordination and good communication with the patient, significant others, where appropriate, and other clinicians. Optimal pharmacotherapy starts with articulation of a working diagnosis and of treatment goals and continues with a plan for ongoing, structured monitoring of symptoms, safety, side effects, adherence, and changes in general health status and psychosocial status. Although progress is being made toward the development of clinically relevant biomarkers and other predictors of drug response, consideration of previous treatment responses, primary and comorbid conditions and symptoms, side-effect profile, drug-drug interactions, and cost often help narrow available treatments to those best suited in a particular clinical context. Beyond selecting appropriate medications and a thoughtful plan for dose titration and monitoring, ensuring that patients has a good understanding of the rationale and plan for treatment and ample opportunity to have questions and concerns addressed at the earliest possible stage in treatment is crucial to medication adherence. For many patients with psychiatric conditions, as with other chronic medical conditions, adherence involves a commitment measured not in days or weeks but in months and years and is core to the success of treatment.

REFERENCES

1. Altshuler L, Suppes T, Black D, et al. Impact of antidepressant discontinuation after acute bipolar depression remission on rates of depressive relapse at 1-year follow-up. Am J Psychiatry 2003;160(7):1252–62.
2. Mander AJ, Loudon JB. Rapid recurrence of mania following abrupt discontinuation of lithium. Lancet 1988;2(8601):15–7.
3. Viguera AC, Whitfield T, Baldessarini RJ, et al. Risk of recurrence in women with bipolar disorder during pregnancy: prospective study of mood stabilizer discontinuation. Am J Psychiatry 2007;164(12):1817–24 [quiz: 1923].
4. Practice guideline for the treatment of patients with major depressive disorder (revision). American Psychiatric Association. Am J Psychiatry 2000;157(Suppl 4): 1–45.
5. Rush AJ, Trivedi MH, Wisniewski SR, et al. Bupropion-SR, sertraline, or venlafaxine-XR after failure of SSRIs for depression. N Engl J Med 2006;354(12):1231–42.
6. Trivedi MH, Fava M, Wisniewski SR, et al. Medication augmentation after the failure of SSRIs for depression. N Engl J Med 2006;354(12):1243–52.
7. Ditto KE. SSRI discontinuation syndrome. Awareness as an approach to prevention. Postgrad Med 2003;114(2):79–84.
8. Alwan S, Friedman JM. Safety of selective serotonin reuptake inhibitors in pregnancy. CNS Drugs 2009;23(6):493–509.
9. Cohen LS, Altshuler LL, Harlow BL, et al. Relapse of major depression during pregnancy in women who maintain or discontinue antidepressant treatment. JAMA 2006;295(5):499–507.

10. Perry R, Cassagnol M. Desvenlafaxine: a new serotonin-norepinephrine reuptake inhibitor for the treatment of adults with major depressive disorder. Clin Ther 2009;31(Pt 1):1374–404.
11. Thase ME. Effects of venlafaxine on blood pressure: a meta-analysis of original data from 3744 depressed patients. J Clin Psychiatry 1998;59(10):502–8.
12. Madhusoodanan S, Bogunovic OJ. Safety of benzodiazepines in the geriatric population. Expert Opin Drug Saf 2004;3(5):485–93.
13. Soumerai SB, Simoni-Wastila L, Singer C, et al. Lack of relationship between long-term use of benzodiazepines and escalation to high dosages. Psychiatr Serv 2003;54(7):1006–11.
14. Wikner BN, Stiller CO, Bergman U, et al. Use of benzodiazepines and benzodi-azepine receptor agonists during pregnancy: neonatal outcome and congenital malformations. Pharmacoepidemiol Drug Saf 2007;16(11):1203–10.
15. Victorri-Vigneau C, Dailly E, Veyrac G, et al. Evidence of zolpidem abuse and dependence: results of the French Centre for Evaluation and Information on Phar-macodependence (CEIP) network survey. Br J Clin Pharmacol 2007;64(2): 198–209.
16. Najjar M. Zolpidem and amnestic sleep related eating disorder. J Clin Sleep Med 2007;3(6):637–8.
17. Hoque R, Chesson AL Jr. Zolpidem-induced sleepwalking, sleep related eating disorder, and sleep-driving: fluorine-18-flourodeoxyglucose positron emission tomography analysis, and a literature review of other unexpected clinical effects of zolpidem. J Clin Sleep Med 2009;5(5):471–6.
18. Zammit G, Erman M, Wang-Weigand S, et al. Evaluation of the efficacy and safety of ramelteon in subjects with chronic insomnia. J Clin Sleep Med 2007;3(5): 495–504.
19. Kanno O, Sasaki T, Watanabe H, et al. Comparison of the effects of zolpidem and triazolam on nocturnal sleep and sleep latency in the morning: a cross-over study in healthy young volunteers. Prog Neuropsychopharmacol Biol Psychiatry 2000; 24(6):897–910.
20. Tondo L, Baldessarini RJ. Long-term lithium treatment in the prevention of suicidal behavior in bipolar disorder patients. Epidemiol Psichiatr Soc 2009; 18(3):179–83.
21. Pinelli JM, Symington AJ, Cunningham KA, et al. Case report and review of the perinatal implications of maternal lithium use. Am J Obstet Gynecol 2002; 187(1):245–9.
22. Yonkers KA, Wisner KL, Stowe Z, et al. Management of bipolar disorder during pregnancy and the postpartum period. Am J Psychiatry 2004;161(4):608–20.
23. Nguyen HT, Sharma V, McIntyre RS. Teratogenesis associated with antibipolar agents. Adv Ther 2009;26(3):281–94.
24. Naber D, Lambert M. The CATIE and CUtLASS studies in schizophrenia: results and implications for clinicians. CNS Drugs 2009;23(8):649–59.
25. Haddad PM, Sharma SG. Adverse effects of atypical antipsychotics: differential risk and clinical implications. CNS Drugs 2007;21(11):911–36.
26. Poulin MJ, Cortese L, Williams R, et al. Atypical antipsychotics in psychiatric practice: practical implications for clinical monitoring. Can J Psychiatry 2005; 50(9):555–62.
27. Mischoulon D. Update and critique of natural remedies as antidepressant treat-ments. Psychiatr Clin North Am 2007;30(1):51–68.
28. Papakostas GI. Evidence for S-adenosyl-L-methionine (SAMe) for the treatment of major depressive disorder. J Clin Psychiatry 2009;70(Suppl 5):18–22.

29. Freeman MP. Omega-3 fatty acids in major depressive disorder. J Clin Psychiatry 2009;70(Suppl 5):7–11.

30. Linde K, Ramirez G, Mulrow CD, et al. St John's wort for depression–an overview and meta-analysis of randomised clinical trials. BMJ 1996;313(7052):253–8.

31. Teschke R, Schwarzenboeck A, Hennermann KH. Kava hepatotoxicity: a clinical survey and critical analysis of 26 suspected cases. Eur J Gastroenterol Hepatol 2008;20(12):1182–93.

32. Birks J, Grimley Evans J. Ginkgo biloba for cognitive impairment and dementia. Cochrane Database Syst Rev 2009;1:CD003120.

An Approach to the Psychosocial Treatment of the Medically Ill Patient

Steven C. Schlozman, MD[a,b,c]

KEYWORDS

• Psychosocial • Coping • Nonpharmacologic • Spiritual

As the practice of medicine becomes increasingly technologically sophisticated and successful in managing and even curing many illnesses, criticisms have arisen that these successes have de-emphasized the less technical aspects of doctoring long thought to characterize good patient care.[1] Chief among these practices are the so-called psychosocial aspects of clinical work. Broadly speaking, these practices include an emphasis on the doctor-patient relationship, the creation of a sound and lasting alliance, and the experience of trust and partnership that the physician fosters in helping the patient to negotiate the complex and uniquely individual experience of being ill.

These criticisms have not been made without considerable thought and study. Patients in Western nations report that they think doctors have a very good grasp of the immense complexity of disease and treatment but, at the same time, are more and more distant from their patients. This is especially ironic given the finding that most medical students continue to apply for medical school with essays that express an overwhelming desire to directly interact with patients in what most would consider a psychosocial setting. In fact, a body of literature now exists that focuses exclusively on how those initially strongly held convictions among medical students are slowly eroded throughout the course of their medical school experience and residency training.[2–4] To suggest that these concerns are entirely a function of the increased capacity to technically heal the sick is inconsistent with existing definitions of doctoring and also not really systemically fair. Very few educators and scholars in medicine would challenge the idea that the art of doctoring includes nonpharmacologic and noninvasive procedures. These skills are every bit as technical (ie, related to technique) as are practices such as prescribing or performing procedures. In

a Medical Student Education in Psychiatry, Harvard Medical School, Boston, MA, USA
b Child and Adolescent Psychiatry Residency, MGH/McLean Program in Child Psychiatry, Boston, MA, USA
c Harvard Graduate School of Education, Massachusetts General Hospital, Yawkey 6900, Boston, MA 02114, USA
E-mail address: sschlozman@partners.org

Med Clin N Am 94 (2010) 1161–1167
doi:10.1016/j.mcna.2010.08.012
0025-7125/10/$ – see front matter © 2010 Elsevier Inc. All rights reserved.

fact, all of these aspects of practicing medicine are intricately intertwined. Additionally, one cannot deny that current market demands emphasize a kind of efficiency that might place at risk some of the more sacred and traditional conceptualizations of being a doctor.[2] Regardless of the possible reasons, however, it seems clear from popular media and evidence-based studies that doctors are being asked by their patients to improve on these less tangible aspects of doctoring.[5]

This article discusses some of these techniques and proposes the argument that unless practitioners of medicine are mindful of the threats to the way they would like and are expected by our patients to practice medicine, they are unlikely to actively endorse changes or to pass the need for these changes onto the next generation of physicians.[5] In this sense, keeping these concerns alive and the subject of ongoing discussion is crucial to the ongoing conceptualization of what it means to be a doctor.

AN HISTORICAL PERSPECTIVE

The romantic image of the doctor on the wards or in the office is ironically at odds with the reality of what most patients experience. Artistic expressions of doctoring, essays about the practice of medicine, and public depictions of working physicians idealize the doctor-patient relationship as central to the therapeutic process or create provocative statements essentially challenging the long-held belief that doctors need to be empathic and caring to be effective. Consider, for example, the stark divide between two separate articles celebrating Norman Rockwell's classic painting depicting a caring visit from the country doctor[6,7] and the average episode of the popular television show "House."[8] These differences serve to accentuate the cognitive dissonance that clinicians and the public experience as each groups tries to glean how best and most effectively to behave with each other.

Also, any attempt to describe the more nuanced aspects of the doctor-patient interaction is to some extent made more difficult by the challenges in defining the nuances themselves.[9] Good nonprocedural and nonpharmacologic care includes widely varying issues from whether one sits or stands[10] to how and with what skills does one develop the art of empathic listening.[11] This article, therefore, attempts to draw from historical conceptualizations of how a doctor ought to behave and to define, as best as possible, whether there is evidence to support intrinsic and measurable value for these often-celebrated behaviors. Central to this thesis is the notion that the role of all doctors in patient care is to help their patients cope as effectively as possible with the realities of being ill.

WHAT IS COPING

Coping is best defined as problem-solving behavior that is intended to bring about relief, reward, quiescence, and equilibrium. Good medical practice calls for the physician to help patients to continually appraise and reappraise the changes in the course of their illness. However, accurate appraisal of coping skills is hampered by muddled definitions of coping, by competing methods of assessment, by a general lack of conscious consideration of how a patient copes, and by uncertainty about whether particular coping styles are effective.[12–15] Currently, most clinicians favor a more open-ended approach to evaluation that considers the unique backgrounds that the patient and the doctor bring to the therapeutic setting.[15]

Additionally, some evidence exists that patients cope better with the understanding that their specialists are highly knowledgeable and not necessarily possessing exemplary bedside manners, whereas patients seem to prefer that their primary care doctors are more willing to make lasting and genuine connections.[16] To this end, the research suggests that different physicians caring for a patient with a complicated problem have differing levels of effectiveness based on the role that they play with the patient. For example, the rare orthopedic consultation need not be nearly as focused on the doctor-patient relationship as the physician who visits a patient multiple times throughout a given course of illness.[16] Having said this, competing views exist, also backed by ample data, that those in seemingly less-connected roles—invasive radiologists, for example—enjoy measurably better patient outcomes when they are respectful in all aspects of patient interaction.[17] Perhaps the simplest conclusion, also borne out by studies of patient satisfaction, is that doctors in general enjoy better outcomes with their patients if they are available, respectful, and seem not to be rushed. A wealth of data supports these guidelines (and it is one of the best defenses against being sued, regardless of whether an error was made in patient care).[18,19]

ENHANCING COPING MECHANISMS

How a person copes depends on the nature of a problem and on the mental, emotional, physical, and social particulars for a given patient, with a special emphasis on the "here and now." Additionally, there are long-established characteristics of those with good and bad coping skills (**Boxes 1** and **2**). These characteristics demonstrate that long- range forays into the past are relevant only if they illuminate the present predicament. In fact, more and more clinicians are adopting a focused and problem-solving approach to therapy with medically ill patients. For example, supportive therapies for medically ill children and adults in both group and individual settings have reduced psychiatric morbidity and had measurable effects on the course of nonpsychiatric illnesses as well.[12,13] There is also increasing support for motivational interviewing (a technique designed to empower patients without patronizing their decisions) as an effective bedside and office tool for better patient outcomes.[20,21]

HELPING PATIENTS ADAPT TO MEDICAL ILLNESS

Adaptation to medical illness is affected by individual, intrahospital, and extrahospital factors.[22] Individual or intrapersonal factors include psychiatric diagnoses (including, but not limited to, depression, anxiety, delirium, dementia, substance abuse,

---

Box 1
Characteristics of those who are good at coping

1. They are optimistic about mastering problems and, despite setbacks, generally maintain a high level of morale.

2. They tend to be practical and to emphasize immediate problems, issues, and obstacles that must be conquered, even before visualizing a remote or ideal resolution.

3. They select from a wide range of potential strategies and tactics, and their policy is not to be at a loss for fallback methods. In this respect, they are resourceful.

4. They heed various possible outcomes and improve coping by being aware of consequences.

5. They are generally flexible and open to suggestions, but they do not give up the final say in decisions.

6. They are composed, although vigilant in avoiding emotional extremes that could impair judgment.

From Schlozman SC, Groves JE, Gross AF, et al. Coping with illness and psychotherapy of the medically ill. In: Stern TA, Fricchione GF, Cassem NH, et al, editors. The MGH hospital of general hospital psychiatry. 6th edition. Philadelphia: Saunders/Elsevier; 2010. p. 425–32; with permission.

Box 2
Characteristics of those who are poor at coping

1. They tend to be excessive in self-expectation, rigid in outlook, inflexible in standards, and reluctant to compromise or to ask for help.

2. Their opinion of how people should behave is narrow and absolute; they allow little room for tolerance.

3. Although prone to firm adherence to preconceptions, they may show unexpected compliance or be suggestible on specious grounds, with little cause.

4. They are inclined to excessive denial and elaborate rationalization; in addition, they are unable to focus on salient problems.

5. Because they find it difficult to weigh feasible alternatives, they tend to be more passive than usual and they fail to initiate action on their own behalf.

6. Their rigidity occasionally lapses, and they subject themselves to impulsive judgments or atypical behavior that fails to be effective.

From Schlozman SC, Groves JE, Gross AF, et al. Coping with illness and psychotherapy of the medically ill. In: Stern TA, Fricchione GF, Cassem NH, et al, editors. The MGH hospital of general hospital psychiatry. 6th edition. Philadelphia: Saunders/Elsevier; 2010. p. 425–32; with permission.

post-traumatic stress disorder, and factitious, somatoform, and sleep disorders). Also, personality style and personality disorders affect how a person copes. Holland and colleagues[23] described the "Five Ds" when discussing what the illness means to a patient: distance (the interruption of interpersonal relationships), dependence (having to rely on others), disability (inability to achieve), disfigurement, and death. Intrahospital factors include the characteristics of the illness (eg, its time course, the intensity of pain, its impact on sleep, surgical interventions, and chemotherapy), whereas extrahospital variables (eg, finances, housing, interpersonal relationships, and sociocultural/language barriers) are also key issues.[22]

Spiritual Concerns

The significance of religious or spiritual conviction in the medically ill deserves special mention. Patients with medical illness face existential issues and, often, crises, as they attempt to glean meaning from their predicament.[24] These concerns are common among patients and present the clinician with an interesting and sometimes unclear set of therapeutic options. Patients may ask "why me," or note that their current circumstances are not "fair." Such ruminations often invoke religious considerations in the patient and the physician; in fact, the medical literature shows a growing appreciation of the important role that can be played by these considerations.[25,26] Because the physician's role involves identification and strengthening of those attributes that are most likely to aid a patient's physical and emotional well-being, effective therapy for the medically ill involves exploring the patient's religious convictions. If religious or spiritual counsel would be of service, attempts should be made to provide this counseling either directly or through pastoral services. It is, however, never the role of the physician to encourage religious conviction de novo, and attempts to do so run the risk of imposing values and beliefs on patients to which they do not adhere, therefore weakening rather than strengthening the alliance.

At the Bedside

In summary, physicians at the bedside have multiple roles. They must combine the complex formulation of disease and treatment with a particular bedside demeanor

> **Box 3**
> **Key questions that can facilitate an alliance and enhance coping and adaptation**
>
> How do you make sense out of your experience?
>
> Who do you believe understands your situation?
>
> What sorts of things keep you from giving up?
>
> Who keeps you alive?
>
> What issues about your treatment concern you the most?
>
> Have there been times when you wanted to give up but did not? What prevented you from giving up?
>
> What things in life are you most grateful for? Has your illness taught you anything meaningful?
>
> *From* Schlozman SC, Groves JE, Gross AF, et al. Coping with illness and psychotherapy of the medically ill. In: Stern TA, Fricchione GF, Cassem NH, et al, editors. The MGH hospital of general hospital psychiatry. 6th edition. Philadelphia: Saunders/Elsevier; 2010. p. 425–32; with permission.

that is consistent with what studies still suggest patients expect from their physicians. The idealized physician continues to be viewed as a kind, calm, and therapeutic individual who engages in shared ownership of the medical problem. This behavior is consistent with better outcomes as well as with what the vast majority of medical students express as a fundamental goal as they enter medicine, and yet, these very descriptors are seen as increasingly lacking in modern health care.[27,28]

This leaves the practicing physician with a major dilemma. There is good evidence that many of the practices that foster connection and healing in the patient-doctor relationship are effective, and yet, these practices were largely developed when the existing milieu allowed one to more easily engage in them. What behavior should practicing physicians pursue to efficiently maximize the goal of helping their patients in the current harried environment?

Studies suggest that fostering a connection with patients does not require inordinate amounts of time and that targeted questions looking at present dilemmas are most effective.[29] **Box 3** outlines some central questions that can be asked at the bedside to facilitate alliance, to increase well-being among patients, and, thus, to assist with coping and adapting to medical illness and hastening recovery.

These questions allow the clinician to succinctly build trust, address meaningful aspects of the patient's illness, and suggest psychological methods by which patients might assist in their recovery. These goals are entirely consistent with the role of the modern doctor and entirely possible even within the current constraints of modern medicine; they enhance patient care and healing and make the practice of medicine infinitely more rewarding and effective.

REFERENCES

1. Dyche L. Interpersonal skill in medicine: the essential partner of verbal communication. J Gen Intern Med 2007;22(7):1035–9.
2. Hojat M, Vergare MJ, Maxwell K, et al. The devil is in the third year: a longitudinal study of erosion of empathy in medical school. Acad Med 2009;84:1182–91 [erratum appears in: Acad Med 2009;84(11):1616].
3. Miles S, Leinster SJ. Identifying professional characteristics of the ideal medical doctor: the laddering technique. Med Teach 2010;32(2):136–91.

4. Winseman J, Malik A, Morison J, et al. Students' views on factors affecting empathy in medical education. Acad Psychiatry 2009;33(6):484–91.
5. Sheth JN, Mittal B. The health of the health care industry: a report card from American consumers. Mark Health Serv 1997;17(4):28–35.
6. Donaldson L. Norman Rockwell visits a family doctor. Clin Med 2002;2(3):266.
7. Schatzki SC. Norman Rockwell visits a country doctor. Am J Roentgenol 1999; 173(4):984.
8. van Mook WN, de Grave WS, Gorter SL, et al. Fellows' in intensive care medicine views on professionalism and how they learn it. Intensive Care Med 2010;36(2):296–303.
9. Frankel RM, Hourigan NT. Thirty-five voices in search of an author: what focus groups reveal about patients experiences in managed care settings. Commun Med 2004;1(1):45–58.
10. Johnson RL, Sadosty AT, Weaver AL, et al. To sit or not to sit? Ann Emerg Med 2008;51(2):188–93,193.e1–2.
11. Anonymous. Patient satisfaction is a best practice. ED Manag 2009;21(10): 114–5.
12. Stauffer MH. A long-term psychotherapy group for children with chronic medical illness. Bull Menninger Clin 1998;62:15–32.
13. Saravay SM. Psychiatric interventions in the medically ill: outcomes and effectiveness research. Psychiatr Clin North Am 1996;19:467–80.
14. Bird B. Talking with patients. 2nd edition. Philadelphia: JB Lippincott; 1973.
15. Coelho G, Hamburg D, Adams J, editors. Coping and adaptation. New York: Basic Books; 1974.
16. Verbeek J, Sengers MJ, Riemens L, et al. Patient expectations of treatment for back pain: a systematic review of qualitative and quantitative studies. Spine 2004;29(20):2309–18.
17. Reynolds A. Patient-centered care. Radiol Technol 2009;81(2):133–47.
18. Rodriguez HP, Rodday AM, Marshall RE, et al. Relation of patients' experiences with individual physicians to malpractice risk. Int J Qual Health Care 2008;20(1):5–12.
19. Stelfox HT, Gandhi TK, Orav EJ, et al. The relation of patient satisfaction with complaints against physicians and malpractice lawsuits. Am J Med 2005; 118(10):1126–33.
20. Anstiss T. Motivational interviewing in primary care. J Clin Psychol Med Settings 2009;16(1):87–93.
21. Meyer C, Muhlfeld A, Drexhage C, et al. Clinical research for patient empowerment–a qualitative approach on the improvement of heart health promotion in chronic illness. Med Sci Monit 2008;14(7):CR358–65.
22. Hunter JJ, Maunder R, Gupta M. Teaching consultation- liaison psychotherapy: assessment of adaptation to medical and surgical illness. Acad Psychiatry 2007;31:367–74.
23. Holland JC, Breitbart W, Jacobsen PB. Psycho-oncology. New York: Oxford University Press; 1998.
24. Schaufel MA, Nordrehaug JE, Malterud K. So you think I'll survive? A qualitative study about doctor-patient dialogues preceding high-risk cardiac surgery or intervention. Heart 2009;95(15):1245–9.
25. Laubmeier KK, Zakowski SG, Bair JP. The role of spirituality in the psychological adjustment to cancer: a test of the transactional model of stress and coping. Int J Behav Med 2004;11(1):48–55.
26. Pargament KI, Koenig HG, Tarakeshwar N, et al. Religious struggle as a predictor of mortality among medically ill patients: a 2-year longitudinal study. Arch Intern Med 2001;161:1881–5.

27. Howe A, Barrett A, Leinster S. How medical students demonstrate their professionalism when reflecting on experience. Med Educ 2009;43(10):942–51.
28. Kind T, Everett VR, Ottolini M. Learning to connect: students' reflections on doctor-patient interactions. Patient Educ Couns 2009;75(2):149–54.
29. Longtin Y, Sax H, Leape LL, et al. Patient participation: current knowledge and applicability to patient safety. Mayo Clin Proc 2010;85(1):53–62.

An Approach to the Patient with Substance Use and Abuse

Jose R. Maldonado, MD[a,b,c,*]

KEYWORDS

• Substance use • Substance abuse • Intoxication • Withdrawal

Substance use is ubiquitous among medically ill patients. A report from the 2008 National Survey on Drug Abuse and Health (NSDAH) sponsored by the Substance Abuse and Mental Health Services Administration estimated 20.1 million Americans aged 12 years or older (8% of the US population) had used an illicit drug (ie, marijuana/hashish, cocaine/crack, heroin, hallucinogens, inhalants, or prescription-type psychotherapeutics used nonmedically) during the month before the survey interview.[1] Marijuana was the most commonly used illicit drug (15.2 million or 6.1%); followed by cocaine (1.9 million, or 0.7%), and hallucinogens (1.1 million, or 0.4%).

Some licit substances also create havoc. The same survey found that slightly more than half (56%) of Americans reported being current drinkers of alcohol; 23.3% participated in binge drinking (ie, ≥ 5 drinks on the same occasion on at least 1 day in the 30 days before the survey), and 6.9% of the population reported heavy drinking (ie, binge drinking on at least 5 days in the past 30 days).[2] Similarly, 6.2 million (2.5%) Americans used prescription-type psychotherapeutic drugs for nonmedical purposes and 70.9 million (or 28.4%) used tobacco during the survey period.

Substance abuse problems were diagnosed in up to 36% of medically hospitalized patients for whom a psychiatric consultation was requested.[3] Therefore, given how prevalent the use of substances is among the medically ill and their potential effect on comorbid medical conditions, it is important for physicians to be mindful of their prevalence and presentation. Because it would be impossible to cover all possible abused substances, this article covers the presenting symptoms of intoxication and withdrawal states, and addresses the acute management of the most commonly

[a] Medicine & Surgery, Stanford University School of Medicine, 401 Quarry Road, Suite #2317, Stanford, CA 94305, USA
[b] Medical & Forensic Psychiatry Section, Stanford University School of Medicine, 401 Quarry Road, Office #2317, Stanford, CA 94305, USA
[c] Psychosomatic Medicine Service, Stanford University School of Medicine, 401 Quarry Road, Office #2317, Stanford, CA 94305, USA
* Medicine & Surgery, Stanford University School of Medicine, 401 Quarry Road, Suite #2317, Stanford, CA 94305.
E-mail address: jrm@stanford.edu

Med Clin N Am 94 (2010) 1169–1205
doi:10.1016/j.mcna.2010.08.010
0025-7125/10/$ – see front matter © 2010 Elsevier Inc. All rights reserved.

medical.theclinics.com

encountered substances (ie, alcohol, nicotine, benzodiazepines [BZs], and opioids), and summarizes all others in a table.

ALCOHOL USE DISORDER
Epidemiology

Ethanol is the second most commonly abused psychotropic drug (after caffeine) and alcohol use disorder (AUD) is the most serious drug abuse problem in the United States[4] and worldwide.[5] According to the Epidemiologic Catchment Area survey, the lifetime prevalence in the general population of alcohol abuse or dependence is 13.6%.[6] Data suggest that alcohol consumption-related problems are the third leading cause of death in the United States.[7] Although alcohol withdrawal is common and usually mild, the abrupt cessation of alcohol consumption by a patient with alcohol dependence may lead to withdrawal seizures or delirium tremens (DTs), either of which may be fatal without adequate treatment.

Although alcoholism is present in 20% to 50% of hospitalized patients, it is diagnosed only about 5% of the time.[8] A poll of physicians affiliated to the American Medical Association revealed that 71% of them believed they were too ambivalent or not competent to properly treat alcoholic patients.[9] Yet, despite the overwhelming statistics, there is still no standardized protocol for the treatment of alcohol withdrawal, and standardized monitoring of patients' withdrawal severity is not common practice.[10]

Mechanism of Action

The effects of alcohol in the central nervous system (CNS) varies and can be divided into acute phase (acute intoxication and early alcohol use) and late stages (development of tolerance and withdrawal syndromes).

Acute stages

Ethanol is the allosteric modulator of γ-aminobutyric acid A ($GABA_A$) receptors. Thus acutely, alcohol renders its central effects (eg, anxiolytic, sedative, anticonvulsant, and motor coordination impairment) mainly through its agonistic effect on $GABA_A$ receptors primarily in the cerebral cortex, medial septal neurons, and hippocampal neurons.[11] In addition, alcohol acutely has a direct inhibitory effect on N-methyl-D-aspartate (NMDA) receptors, thus reducing excitatory glutamatergic transmission.[12] It also disinhibits GABA-mediated dopaminergic-projections to the ventral tegmental area (VTA), leading to increases in extracellular dopamine (DA) in the nucleus accumbens (NA), which are likely responsible for the initially pleasurable effects of alcohol and for the impulse to drink more.[13]

Late stages

The development of alcohol tolerance with chronic ethanol use is a neuroadaptive process (to reduce the acute effects of alcohol and provide homeostasis). Thus, chronic alcohol intake leads to an adaptive suppression of GABA activity, mediated by internalization and downregulation of $GABA_A$-BZ receptor complexes.[14] Chronic alcohol consumption also leads to increased synaptic glutamate (GLU) release, as well as increased NMDA and non-NMDA (eg, α-amino-3-hydroxy-5-methyl-4-isoxazolepropionic acid receptor [AMPA], kainate receptors, and voltage-gated Ca^{++} channels) glutamatergic receptor activity. In addition, chronic ethanol exposure (habituation) leads to overactivity of noradrenergic neurons in the CNS[15–17] and the peripheral nervous system[17,18] likely via desensitization of α_2 receptors or lack of α_2 agonist activity and excessive norepinephrine (NE) production as the excess extracellular DA is converted into NE via DA-β-hydroxylase.

During alcohol withdrawal syndromes (AWSs), excess noradrenergic activity leads to the development of autonomic hyperactivity (eg, anxiety, tremor, sweating, hypertension, tachycardia).[15,17,19] Examination of cerebrospinal fluid reveals that GABA levels are low[12] whereas GLU[20] 3-methoxy-4-hydrophenylglycol (MHPG)[15,19] levels are increased in patients undergoing alcohol withdrawal. Data suggest that an increase in plasma free-MHPG concentration may similarly play a role in the evolution of delirium from nonalcohol withdrawal causes,[21] suggesting that these 2 types of delirium may have a common pathway in dysregulation of the catecholamine system.[22] Similarly, the reduction in GABA-ergic neuronal transmission and an increase in glutamatergic transmission during alcohol withdrawal may lead to CNS hyperexcitation and the development of seizures.[23]

Acute Alcohol Intoxication

The effect of the patient's blood alcohol level (BAL) depends on whether the patient is habituated to alcohol. Nonhabituated individuals experience increased CNS depression as the BAL escalates, going from mild problems of coordination and euphoria, to poor judgment and impaired reaction time, to anesthesia, to unconsciousness, to coma, to death as a result of respiratory depression (**Fig. 1**).

Management of Acute Alcohol Intoxication

There is no specific treatment of acute alcohol intoxication. The immediate steps for management include a complete assessment of the patient's medical status, including acute and long-term sequelae of alcohol use and current respiratory status; exploration of intoxication with other possible substances that may aggravate the patient's CNS status; and prophylaxis against possible withdrawal (**Box 1**). There is no evidence that gastric lavage or activated charcoal are of benefit.

Otherwise, the management of acute intoxication is primarily supportive. If an alteration of mental status is observed the blood glucose level should be checked, and if low, a dextrose infusion administered. To prevent Wernicke encephalopathy parenteral thiamine should be administered along with glucose. Patients with mild intoxication are likely to require little more than appropriate fluids and nutrition and a safe place to get sober. Patients with moderate intoxication may require vitamin and parenteral fluid replacement, monitoring of vital signs and mental status, and monitoring for the possible development of withdrawal syndromes. Depending on the patient's history, initiation of a withdrawal protocol may be required. In mental status changes that seem in excess to the BAL, brain imaging may be required to rule out intracranial processes, from concussions to subdural hematomas.

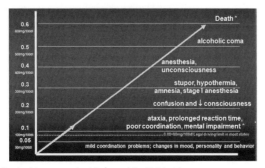

Fig. 1. Effects of alcohol in a nonhabituated individual.

> **Box 1**
> **Management of acute alcohol intoxication**
>
> There is no antidote for alcohol intoxication. Treatment is supportive and symptomatic, it includes:
>
> 1. Assessment of respiratory status and determination on whether intubation for airway protection is required
>
> 2. Metabolic assessment; including electrolyte, glucose, and fluid status
>
> 3. Before glucose is administered, consider supplementation with thiamine, to prevent Wernicke-Korsakoff syndrome
>
> 4. Toxicology assessment, to determine whether other substances may contribute to the patient's condition; the presence of other CNS-depressant agents (eg, BZs, barbiturates, opioids) may increase the risk for respiratory depression, need for intubation, delirium, and withdrawal syndromes
>
> 5. The overall management of acute intoxication depends on the patient's degree of habituation, the total amount of alcohol ingested, and the presence of other ingested substances
>
>   a. Most patients with mild to moderate intoxication do well with minimal treatment
>
>   b. Patients with severe intoxication may require further observation and possibly endotracheal intubation for airway protection

Patients with severe intoxication may require observation (of mental status, vital signs, and respiratory status). In some patients, prophylactic intubation for airway protection may be appropriate.

AWSs

AWSs occur after a period of absolute or, in some cases, relative abstinence from alcohol. Therefore, it is possible for patients to experience an AWS even although they may have a high BAL. Typically, AWS begin within 6 to 24 hours after alcohol cessation or decreased intake in habituated individuals (**Fig. 2**).

Early Withdrawal (the Shakes)

Tremors begin on the first day, peaking about 16 to 24 hours (in 90% of cases) after a relative or absolute abstinence from alcohol. At times the onset may be as late as 10 days after the last drink. Tremors, nervousness, irritability, nausea, and vomiting are the earliest and most common signs. Tremors are usually generalized, coarse, and of fast frequency (about 5–7 cycles/s) and they worsen with motor activity or emotional stress. Once begun, the syndrome varies in duration and severity. In

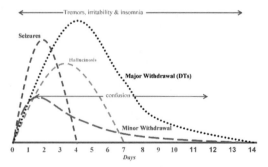

Fig. 2. Alcohol withdrawal/abstinence syndromes.

uncomplicated cases, withdrawal usually subsides in 5 to 7 days even without treatment. Symptoms (eg, anorexia, nausea, vomiting, psychological tension, general malaise, hypertension, autonomic hyperactivity, tachycardia, diaphoresis, orthostatic hypotension, irritability, vivid dreams, and insomnia) may last up to 14 days. Extrapyramidal symptoms may occur during alcohol withdrawal after several weeks of continuous drinking or after an intensive brief binge of a day's duration, even in a patient not previously or currently treated with antipsychotics.

Alcohol Withdrawal Seizures (Rum Fits)

Withdrawal seizures begin on the first day, peaking about 12 to 48 hours (95% occurring within 7–38 hours) after a relative or absolute abstinence from alcohol. Grand mal seizures arise in up to 25% of patients with an AWS and are characterized by generalized seizures that occur during the course of alcohol withdrawal, usually in the absence of an underlying seizure disorder. Several metabolic abnormalities are associated with their occurrence, including low serum Mg^{++}, respiratory alkalosis, hypoglycemia, and increased intracellular sodium. About one-third of patients who develop alcohol withdrawal seizures experience only one seizure, whereas two-thirds have multiple seizures, often closely spaced, if untreated. Only a few (about 2%) develop status epilepticus, most often patients with epilepsy who have stopped their anticonvulsant prescriptions. The presence of seizures has important prognostic value in predicting a complicated withdrawal period because about one-third of patients who develop seizures go on to develop secondary DTs.

Alcoholic Hallucinosis

Hallucinosis often begins on the first day, peaking about 48 to 96 hours after a relative or absolute abstinence from alcohol. Alcoholic hallucinations usually consist of primarily auditory (or less frequently visual) misperceptions. By definition, the sensorium is clear and vital signs are stable, differentiating it from DTs; some signs of early withdrawal may be present. The time to resolution is a few hours to days. Hallucinations may persist after all other withdrawal symptoms have resolved.

DTs

DTs usually appear 1 to 3 days after a relative or absolute abstinence from alcohol. The peak intensity usually occurs on the fourth to fifth day after abstinence. It occurs in up to 10% of alcoholics hospitalized for detoxification. Its mortality is high: about 1% in treated cases and up to 15% when left untreated. When DTs co-occur with certain medical conditions, mortality may increase to 20%. DTs are differentiated from uncomplicated withdrawal by the presence of a profound confusional state (ie, delirium). Symptoms commonly include confusion, disorientation, a fluctuating or clouded consciousness, perceptual disturbances (eg, auditory or visual hallucinations or illusions), agitation, insomnia, fever, and autonomic hyperactivity. Terror, agitation, and primarily visual (sometimes tactile) hallucinations of insects, small animals, or other perceptual distortions can also occur. The confusion and mental status changes can last from a few days to a several weeks, even after resolution of the physical symptoms of withdrawal. Most cases subside after 3 days of severe DTs followed by minor symptoms that may last as long as 5 weeks. DT-related deaths are usually the result of medical complications (eg, infections, cardiac arrhythmias, fluid and electrolyte abnormalities, pyrexia, poor hydration, hypertension, or suicide in response to hallucinations or delusions).

Alcohol Withdrawal Treatment

The effective management of AWS includes a combination of supportive and pharmacologic measures. Supportive measures include the stabilization and management of concurrent medical problems, cessation of all alcohol intake, and use of nutritional supplementation (**Box 2**).

The pharmacologic management of AWS has been a source of controversy. The use of alcohol replacement and barbiturates used to be the norm; more recently, BZs have been favored.[24–27] A Cochrane review, including 57 trials and 4051 subjects, showed that BZs offered a large benefit against AWS (particularly seizures when compared with placebo).[28]

Once the diagnosis of AWS has been made and other medical complications are being corrected, objective tools (eg, the Clinical Institute Withdrawal Assessment for Alcohol-Revised [CIWA-Ar] Scale (**Fig. 3**),[29] and the Alcohol-Withdrawal Syndrome Scale [AWSS] to assess the severity of the AWS) should be used (**Fig. 4**).[30]

Mild withdrawal (CIWA-Ar ≤8) (AWSS ≤5) may require no treatment. If the patient has no history of alcohol withdrawal and has a history of moderate alcohol consumption, observation with symptomatic treatment (eg, diazepam 5–10 mg by mouth every 6–8 hours, as needed) may suffice.

Moderate withdrawal (CIWA-Ar >8–15) (AWSS 6–9) should be treated based on a withdrawal management protocol (ie, loading vs symptom-triggered method). The goal is to have a patient who is comfortable (and arousable) and with stable vital signs.

Severe withdrawal (CIWA-Ar >15) (AWSS ≥10) requires aggressive treatment based on a withdrawal management protocol (ie, loading vs symptom-triggered method). Patients in severe withdrawal may require treatment in a monitored bed with intravenous sedation. BZ doses should be repeated until symptomatic relief and light sedation have been achieved. The goal is to have a patient who is comfortable (and arousable) with stable vital signs.

Alcohol withdrawal management protocol

Clinicians have been divided between 2 main treatment methods. The loading method (**Box 3**) requires the use of a long-acting agent (eg, diazepam, chlordiazepoxide), thus allowing for loading of the agents, followed by slow elimination (linked to its long half-life). Conversely, the symptom-triggered method (**Box 4**) advocates for the use of short-acting agents (eg, lorazepam) and allows for multiple doses based on the need (ie, symptoms) as measured by an objective withdrawal scale.

A recent study by Maldonado and colleagues[25] failed to reveal a clinical advantage for choosing a BZ according to their half-lives (eg, lorazepam vs diazepam); no statistically significant difference was found in 4 key measures: reduction in duration of symptoms (as measured by CIWA-Ar or AWSS scores); normalization of sympathetic activity (as measured by systolic blood pressure [SBP]); length of hospital stay; or total BZ usage. Nevertheless, nursing staff preferred the loading method because of ease of administration and less irritability in patients on long-acting agents. Yet, recent reviews point toward longer-acting agents for superior prevention of alcohol-related seizures.[27,31]

Adjunctive Treatment of Alcohol Withdrawal

Antipsychotic agents

Practice guidelines from the American Society of Addiction Medicine has advised against the use of neuroleptic agents as the sole pharmacologic agents in the setting of DTs, as they are associated with a longer duration of delirium, higher complication rates and, ultimately, higher mortality.[27] The addition of typical (eg, haloperidol) or second-generation (eg, olanzapine) antipsychotics as needed may be useful in

---

Box 2
Basic management of alcohol withdrawal

- Stabilize the patient

    Before initiating any specific treatment of alcohol withdrawal, perform a thorough assessment of the patient's medical condition; particularly looking for the acute (ie, dehydration, subdural hematoma, Mallory-Weiss tears, gastritis) and long-term (eg, alcoholic cirrhosis, malnutrition) sequelae of alcohol abuse

    Correct fluid, electrolyte, and nutritional deficiencies

- Toxicology

    Obtain a complete toxicology screening test, which may help assess the patient's starting BAL, but also look for the possibility of other substances that may complicate the picture; the concurrent abuse of other CNS-depressant substances (eg, barbiturates, BZs) may lead to more a complicated, and more difficult-to-treat AWS; likewise, the presence of a CNS stimulant may predict agitation or psychosis early in the course of treatment

    BAL on admission

- Urine toxicology screening tests on admission and as needed

- Total abstinence from alcohol

- Avoid all alcohol use; there is no scientific evidence showing the usefulness of alcohol by mouth in the management of alcohol withdrawal

- Specific measures:

    Correct and monitor fluid balances, electrolytes, and vital signs.

    Vitamin supplementation:

    　Thiamine 100 mg intravenously/intramuscularly/by mouth × 3 to 5 days

    　Folate 1 mg by mouth daily

    　Multivitamin, 1 tab by mouth daily

    　B complex vitamin 2 tabs by mouth daily

    　Vitamin K 5 to 10 mg subcutaneously × 1 (if international normalized ratio [INR] is >1.3)

    Monitor:

    　Vital signs every 2 hours

    　Blood glucose level

    　Fluid balance

    　Electrolytes (especially Mg^{++}, Na^+, K^+)

- Behavioral management:

    Frequent and appropriate reality orientation

    Adequate maintenance of sleep/wake cycle; keep patients in a tranquil, well-lit space during daytime; lights off at night

    Restraints may be needed for combative/agitated patients

    Sitters may be required for patients who are confused or in restraints

---

severely agitated patients or in those experiencing severe hallucinosis unresponsive to BZs. If these agents are to be used, they should always be added after adequate treatment of withdrawal symptoms with BZs, because they may help to control the agitation, but do not cross-cover the effect of other CNS-depressant agents.

FIGURE 1

The Clinical Institute Withdrawal Assessment for Alcohol—Revised

Addiction Research Foundation Clinical Institute Withdrawal Assessment for Alcohol (CIWA-Ar)

Patient _____   Date |—|—|—| Time ____:____
                                                    Y m d   (24-hour clock, midnight=00:00)

Pulse or heart rate, taken for one minute: _____   Blood pressure: _____ / _____

NAUSEA AND VOMITING—Ask "Do you feel sick to your stomach? Have you vomited?" Observation.
0 no nausea and no vomiting
1 mild nausea with no vomiting
2
3
4 intermittent nausea with dry heaves
5
6
7 constant nausea, frequent dry heaves and vomiting

TREMOR—Arms extended and fingers spread apart. Observation.
0 no tremor
1 not visible, but can be felt fingertip to fingertip
2
3
4 moderate, with patient's arm extended
5
6
7 severe, even with arms not extended

PAROXYSMAL SWEATS—Observation.
0 no sweat visible
1 barely perceptible sweating, palms moist
2
3
4 beads of sweat obvious on forehead
5
6
7 drenching sweats

ANXIETY—Ask "Do you feel nervous?" Observation.
0 no anxiety, at ease
1 mildly anxious
2
3
4 moderately anxious, or guarded, so anxiety is inferred
5
6
7 equivalent to acute panic states as seen in severe delirium
   or acute schizophrenic reactions

AGITATION—Observation.
0 normal scarcity
1 somewhat more than normal activity
2
3
4 moderately fidgety and restless
5
6
7 paces back and forth during most of the interview,
   or constantly thrashes about

TACTILE DISTURBANCES—Ask "Have you any itching, pins and needles sensations, any burning, any numbness, or do you feel bugs crawling on or under your skin?" Observation.
0 none
1 very mild itching, pins and needles, burning or numbness
2 mild itching, pins and needles, burning or numbness
3 moderate itching, pins and needles, burning or numbness
4 moderately severe hallucinations
5 severe hallucinations
6 extremely severe hallucinations
7 continuous hallucinations

AUDITORY DISTURBANCES—Ask "Are you more aware of sounds around you? Are they harsh? Do they frighten you? Are you hearing anything that is disturbing to you? Are you hearing things you know are not there?" Observation.
0 not present
1 very mild harshness or ability to frighten
2 mild harshness or ability to frighten
3 moderate harshness or ability to frighten
4 moderately severe hallucinations
5 severe hallucinations
6 extremely severe hallucinations
7 continuous hallucinations

VISUAL DISTURBANCES—Ask "Does the light appear to be too bright? Is its color different? Does it hurt your eyes? Are you seeing anything that is disturbing to you? Are you seeing things you know are not there?" Observation.
0 not present
1 very mild sensitivity
2 mild sensitivity
3 moderate sensitivity
4 moderately severe hallucinations
5 severe hallucinations
6 extremely severe hallucinations
7 continuous hallucinations

HEADACHE, FULLNESS IN HEAD—Ask "Does your head feel different? Does it feel like there is a band around your head?" Do not rate for dizziness or lightheadedness. Otherwise, rate severity.
0 not present
1 very mild
2 mild
3 moderate
4 moderately severe
5 severe
6 very severe
7 extremely severe

ORIENTATION AND CLOUDING OF SENSORIUM—Ask "What day is this? Where are you? Who am I?"
0 oriented and can do serial additions
1 cannot do serial additions or is uncertain about date
2 disoriented for date by no more than 2 calendar days
3 disoriented for date by more than 2 calendar days
4 disoriented for place and/or person

This scale is not copyrighted and may be used freely.

Total CIWA-Ar Score ____
Rater's Initials ____
Maximum Possible Score 67

Fig. 3. The CIWA-Ar.

β-Adrenergic Blockers

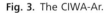

β-Blockers reduce autonomic manifestations of acute alcohol withdrawal.[27] Although these medications relieve autonomic hyperactivity, they do not mitigate the CNS effects, such as seizures or hallucinosis. Certain β-blockers (eg, propranolol) have been associated with a higher incidence of delirium and should be avoided.[32] Therefore, these agents should be used in conjunction with BZs to treat autonomic hyperactivity (eg, atenolol 50 mg by mouth daily for heart rate >80 beats/min) after appropriate coverage with a BZ has been achieved.

Patient Name:
MR#:
Date:
Time:

Somatic (S) Subscale: Somatic symptoms					
Score →	0	1	2	3	Total ↓
Pulse rate/min	<100	101 – 110	111 – 120	>120	
Diastolic BP (mmHg)	<95	96 – 100	101 – 105	>105	
Temperature (°C)	<37.0	37.0 – 37.5	37.6 – 38.0	>38.0	
Respiratory rate/min	<20	20 – 24	>24		
Perspiration	None	Mild (wet hands)	Moderate (forehead)	Severe (profuse)	
Tremor	None	Mild (arms raised & finger spread)	Moderate (fingers spread)	Severe (spontaneous)	
				Sub score of somatic symptoms →	

Mental (M) Subscale: Mental symptoms						
Score →	0	1	2	3	4	Total ↓
Agitation	None	Restless	Rolling in bed	Try to leave bed	In rage	
Contact	Short talk possible	Easily distractible	Drifting contact	Dialogue impossible		
Orientation (time, place, person, situation)	Fully aware	One sphere disturbed	Two spheres disturbed	Totally confused		
Hallucinations	None	Uncertain	One kind present	Two kinds present	All kinds	
Anxiety	None	Mild (only if asked)	Severe (spontaneous complaint)			
				Sub score of mental symptoms →		
Total score T = S + M →						

Original text: Wetterling et.al., 1997[30].

Legend:

Classification	AWS Score
Mild AWS	≤ 5
Moderate	6 – 9
Severe AWS	≥ 10

Fig. 4. AWSS. (*Adapted from* Wetterling T, Kanitz RD, Besters B, et al. A new rating scale for the assessment of the alcohol-withdrawal syndrome (AWS scale). Alcohol Alcohol 1997;32:756; with permission.)

Potential Alternative Treatments for Alcohol Withdrawal

Anticonvulsants

The routine use of phenytoin in cases of alcohol withdrawal seizures is controversial. A meta-analysis of randomized, placebo-controlled trials for the secondary prevention of alcohol withdrawal seizures showed lorazepam to be effective in contrast to phenytoin.[33] The data do not indicate that anticonvulsants are needed for the prophylaxis of alcohol withdrawal seizures in the average alcoholic, although they may have a role in patients at high risk for alcohol withdrawal seizures.

Yet, new promising data on the use of carbamazepine are emerging.[34,35] Randomized double-blind controlled trials (ie, carbamazepine vs BZs) have found that both drugs were equally efficacious in treating AWS, yet carbamazepine had greater efficacy in preventing posttreatment relapses to drinking and greater reduction of anxiety symptoms.[34,35] A Cochrane database systematic review suggested that carbamazepine had a small but statistically significant protective effect over BZ.[36] Oxcarbazepine, an analogue of carbamazepine, has shown comparable effects to carbamazepine in the treatment of AWS in several studies,[37] including relapse prevention.[38]

Box 3
Management of alcohol withdrawal: BZ loading method

This method requires the use of a long-acting agent (eg, diazepam, chlordiazepoxide), which is administered until there has been significant improvement in withdrawal symptoms. It is postulated that agents with long half-lives allow for self-tapering of the drug, which translates into ease of administration and avoidance of breakthrough symptoms caused by undersedation. Critics of this method highlight the possibility of oversedation, which may result in respiratory depression and prolonged hospitalizations.

Mild withdrawal (CIWA-Ar ≤8) (AWSS ≤5):

   May require no treatment

   If the patient has no history of significant alcohol withdrawal and has a history of moderate alcohol consumption, observation with symptomatic treatment (eg, diazepam 5–10 mg by mouth every 6–8 hours, as needed) may be enough

Moderate withdrawal (CIWA-Ar >8–15) (AWSS 6–9):

   Diazepam 20 mg, by mouth, every 1 hour × 3

   Stop the loading if the patient becomes hypersomnolent, is difficult to arouse, or has signs of respiratory depression

   The average required doses range between 60 and 120 mg (total loading) for patients with DTs alone; the required dose may be higher in patients with significant tolerance or combined alcohol and BZ/barbiturate dependence

   Infrequently, additional doses may be needed at bedtime to supplement initial loading and/or treat insomnia

Complicated withdrawal (CIWA-Ar >15) (AWSS ≥10):

   Diazepam 20 mg, by mouth/intravenously, repeat every 30 to 60 minutes until the patient is sedated but arousable

   The average required doses range between 60 and 160 mg (total loading) for patients with DTs alone and between 60 and 215 mg if there are other medical illnesses as well. The required dose may be higher in patients with significant tolerance or combined alcohol and BZ/barbiturate dependence

   Stop the loading if the patient becomes hypersomnolent, is difficult to arouse, or has signs of respiratory depression

   Infrequently, additional doses may be needed at bedtime to supplement initial loading and/or treat insomnia; once withdrawal symptoms have abated, the long half-life of diazepam may allow for a smooth self-taper

   • For mild reemergence of withdrawal symptoms:

      Give diazepam (Valium) 10–25 mg by mouth at bedtime

      Taper smaller doses over a period of 1 to 2 weeks

In severe liver disease, patients with compromised hepatic function, and in elderly patients, consider short to intermediate-acting (half-life) agents. Lorazepam (and oxazepam) offers alternate hepatic metabolism and has no active metabolites.

In a recent placebo-controlled study, both lamotrigine and topiramate significantly reduced observer-rated and self-rated withdrawal severity, dysphoric mood, and supplementary diazepam administration when compared with placebo; they were as effective as diazepam.[39] Other drugs for which there is limited evidence for the treatment of AWS are gabapentin,[40] pregabalin,[41,42] tiagabine,[43] and vigabatrin.[44]

Box 4
Management of alcohol withdrawal: symptom-triggered method

The second symptom-triggered method promotes the use of short-acting agents (eg, lorazepam) administered in accordance with regular symptom monitoring (eg, CIWA-Ar).[29] A recent study using this symptom-triggered model reported a shorter time to symptom control and a total lower medication needed, compared with a nonprotocol infusion method. Proponents of this method suggest that it prevents oversedation which in turn translates into faster resolution of symptoms and earlier discharge from hospital. Critics highlight problems of breakthrough withdrawal, the need for constant monitoring and frequent medication administration, and a potentially greater problem with the development of benzodiazepine dependence.

Mild withdrawal (CIWA-Ar ≤8)(AWSS ≤5):

  May require no treatment

  If the patient has no history of significant alcohol withdrawal and has a history of moderate alcohol consumption, observation with symptomatic treatment (eg, lorazepam 1–2 mg by mouth every 4–6 hours, as needed) may be enough

Moderate (CIWA-Ar = 9–15) and severe withdrawal (CIWA-Ar >15) (AWSS >6)):

  Lorazepam (Ativan) 2 mg intravenously/by mouth every 1 to 2 hours, as needed

  Repeat doses until sedation has been achieved

  Once symptoms are under control and the CIWA-Ar ≤8 for 24 hours, begin to taper lorazepam by 25% of original 24-hour requirement per day until off

  Stop the loading if the patient becomes hypersomnolent, is difficult to arouse, or has signs of respiratory depression

  The required dose may be higher in patients with significant tolerance or combined alcohol and BZ/barbiturate dependence

  Infrequently additional doses may be needed at bedtime to supplement initial loading and/or treat insomnia

  These guidelines should be used in patients with hepatic dysfunction (INR >1.6); renal insufficiency (CrCl <30 mL/min, SCr >2); or head trauma (in whom frequent CNS assessments are required)

α₂ *Adrenergic Receptor Agonists*

Given our current understanding of the effects of chronic alcohol use on the CNS and the effects of AWS on the catecholamine system one should consider the potential use of α_2 agonists in the management of AWS.[45] When compared with BZs, clonidine has been more effective in the management of physiologic hyperactivity as measured by objective withdrawal criteria (eg, heart rate, blood pressure), psychological symptoms (eg, anxiety, irritability, agitation), and CNS excitation (ie, seizures, DTs) associated with alcohol withdrawal.[46,47]

Similarly, the new α_2 adrenergic agonist, dexmedetomidine, may prove equally efficacious in the management of AWS. Laboratory data, in rats, have shown its efficacy in managing all phases of AWS.[48] Several clinical reports suggest dexmedetomidine has been efficacious when BZs have failed to effectively manage AWS.[49–51]

All physicians treating patients with active AWS have had patients with protracted delirium or confusional states even well after the physiologic instability has resolved. Even although some of these states may be the sequelae of having experienced AWS, delirium and cognitive impairment may be mediated by the choice of therapeutic agent. Some studies have suggested that BZs may be associated with the development of delirium.[52] Others have found that BZ use (and its amount) is an independent risk factor for the development of delirium.[22,53–55]

Maldonado and colleagues[56] showed that avoiding the use of GABA-ergic agents (ie, BZs and propofol) by using dexmedetomidine, as an alternative for sedation, was associated with a significant decrease in the development of postoperative delirium. Thus, at least in some patients, the use of alternative agents (ie, non-BZs) may help in controlling the autonomic manifestations of AWS, reduce agitation, and some of the other behavioral manifestations of AWS (eg, anxiety) and should be considered as an adjunct to, and possibly even as alternative to, conventional BZ management. Caution in its use as a single agent should be exercised until further head-to-head studies with BZs have been conducted and their efficacy in preventing seizures has been shown.

Management of Alcohol Dependence

A comprehensive description of the long-term management of alcohol dependence is beyond the scope of this review and has been described in detail elsewhere.[57–59] The ultimate goal is to assist patients resume a normal level of function and to promote alcohol abstinence. Nonpharmacologic interventions that have proved successful include cognitive behavioral therapy (CBT),[60] motivational interviewing,[61] and the brief physician intervention model promoted by the National Institute for Alcohol Abuse and Alcoholism.[62] Studies have found that the combination of psychotherapy and medication was superior to either approach alone.[63,64] Alcoholics Anonymous meetings are the most widespread and available treatment, but research data regarding its efficacy are lacking.[65]

Currently, 3 medications are approved by the US Food and Drug Administration (FDA) for the treatment of alcohol dependence. Disulfiram, an aldehyde dehydrogenase inhibitor, causes the classic antabuse reaction (ie, palpitations, flushing, hypotension, tachycardia, headache, nausea, and vomiting) when patients treated with disulfiram drink alcohol, caused by a fast accumulation of acetaldehyde (aversive technique).[66] Open-label studies have suggested that disulfiram may be superior to acamprosate[67] and naltrexone[68] in preventing alcohol abuse relapse. Severe adverse psychiatric and medical reactions (eg, myocardial infarction, congestive heart failure, respiratory depression, and convulsions), including death, have been associated with its use.[69] Acamprosate,[70] a structural analogue of GABA and GLU, is believed to interact with these neurotransmitter systems in the CNS to attenuate glutamatergic excitation that occurs with abstinence and thus to reduce alcohol craving.[2,71] Despite initially encouraging results, the data are mixed regarding its efficacy.[72] Naltrexone, an opiate receptor antagonist, blocks the reinforcing effects of alcohol by preventing the stimulation of opioid receptors and the reduction of DA release in the VTA.[73] Some large studies have contradicted their efficacy for alcohol dependence.[72]

There are a few pharmacologic treatments not approved by the FDA. Topiramate, an anticonvulsant, has been widely used in the treatment of disorders characterized by impulsivity and studies have suggested that it reduces drinking, probably by behavioral inhibition.[74,75] Gabapentin, an anticonvulsant, has significantly greater reductions (than placebo) on several measures of subjective craving for alcohol as well as for evoked craving, and its use was associated with significant improvement on several measures of sleep quality.[76] Pregabalin, an anticonvulsant, has the same range of efficacy as naltrexone regarding drinking indices and craving scores, yet patients treated with pregabalin reported greater improvement of specific symptoms (eg, anxiety, hostility, psychoticism, survival function).[77] Baclofen, a muscle relaxant, may alleviate AWS and craving through inhibition of DA and GLU release, showing some promise in small studies and case reports,[78] although failing to compare favorably with BZs.[79] Ondansetron, a 5-hydroxytryptamine-3 (5-HT$_3$)-receptor antagonist, reduces alcohol consumption by decreasing alcohol cue-induced activation of the ventral striatum.[80] Preliminary findings suggest that ondansetron may be effective in the treatment of early-onset alcoholics, who respond poorly to psychosocial treatment alone, although the drug does not seem to work well in other types of alcoholics.[81]

OPIOIDS
Epidemiology

In 2008, 453,000 Americans aged 12 years and older had abused heroin at least once in the year before being surveyed.[1] Americans constitute 4.6% of the world's population, but consume approximately 80% of the world's opiates.[82] In 2008, there were 114,000 persons aged 12 years or older who had used heroin for the first time within the past 12 months.[1] Prescription opioids have been considered an important gateway drug, and the fact that they are prescribed by doctors lulls users into believing they are safe. Studies suggest that drug dealers are a small source of illicitly used prescription opioids. Diversion through family and friends is now the greatest source of illicit opioids. Data also suggest that most of these opioids are obtained from a single physician, not from doctor shopping.[1]

Mechanism of Action

There are 5 types of opioid receptors in mammals: μ, κ, σ, δ, and ε subtypes.[83] These subtypes are located in the periaqueductal gray area of brain, spinal cord, peripheral nerves, adrenal medulla, ganglia, and gut. Stimulation of μ and σ receptors produces intense feelings of well-being and euphoria. The dopaminergic mesolimbic system, which originates in the VTA of the midbrain and projects to the NA, is crucial in the reward effects of intracranial self-stimulation, the natural rewards of water and food intake, and the action of drugs of abuse, including opioids. Basal activity of this system, expressed in DA release in the NA, is under the tonic control of opposing opioid systems, activation of μ- and σ-receptors increases, whereas κ-receptor activation decreases the basal activity of the mesolimbic system.

Opiates, like heroin, modify the action of DA in the NA and the VTA, part of the brain's reward pathway. Once it has crossed the blood-brain barrier, heroin is converted to morphine, a powerful agonist at the μ opioid receptors subtype. This binding inhibits the release of GABA, thus reducing the inhibitory effect of GABA on dopaminergic neurons. The increased activation of dopaminergic neurons and subsequent release of DA results in sustained activation of the postsynaptic membrane, leading to the feelings of euphoria and the high associated with opiate use.[83] New emerging evidence suggests that activation of μ opioid receptor significantly inhibits the glutamatergic excitatory postsynaptic currents in the anterior cingulate cortex neurons, via suppression of presynaptic GLU release.[84]

Opioid Intoxication

Opioid intoxication is suspected when patients present with symptoms of opioid effect (particularly depressed mental status) and confirmation with toxicology tests or evidence of opioid overdose (eg, empty bottles, suicide note). A useful mnemonic to remember the effects of opioid agents is MORPHINE-ABC (**Box 5**). Data suggest that most deaths related to the use of prescription opioids occur in conjunction with

---

Box 5
Signs of opioid intoxication: MORPHINE-ABC

Miosis

Out of it (sedation)

Respiratory depression and decreased tidal volume

Pneumonia (aspiration)

Hypotension/hypothermia

Infrequency (constipation, decreased bowel sounds, urinary retention)

Nausea

Emesis/euphoria

Analgesia

Bradycardia

Coma (or altered mental status)

---

one or more widely available and legally dispensed nonopioid, CNS-depressant substances (eg, alcohol, BZs, cyclic antidepressants).[85]

Management of Acute Intoxication

Treatment includes discontinuation of opiates (eg, surreptitious drug use, removal of transdermal delivery system), use of supportive measures (eg, respiratory rate, temperature, hydration), treatment of other medical problems (eg, infections, head injury), and the administration of an opioid antagonist. Special attention is also required when there is a possibility of multiple drug intoxication (eg, suicidal overdose) because some substances, particularly CNS depressants, may potentiate the respiratory suppressant effect of opioids. Some agents have specific toxicities, such as serotonin syndrome (ie, meperidine), seizure (eg, meperidine, propoxyphene, tramadol), hepatotoxicity (especially with opioid compounds containing acetaminophen), and cardiac dysrryhtmias (ie, methadone has been associated with QTC prolongation; propoxyphene with QRS prolongation), which need special attention from health providers. The treatment of choice for acute intoxication is the administration of an opioid antagonist (ie, naloxone) (**Table 1**).[86]

Management of Opioid Withdrawal

The time to onset of opioid withdrawal symptoms depends on the half-life of the substance being used. For the most part, the symptoms of opioid withdrawal are uncomfortable, but seldom life-threatening (**Table 2**). The reintroduction of an opioid most certainly alleviates or eliminates most withdrawal symptoms. To achieve this, substitute agents are often temporarily used for detoxification. In the United States, the choices of agents include a long-acting opioid (eg, methadone)[88] or a partial μ-opioid receptor agonist and κ-opioid receptor antagonist (ie, buprenorphine, a partial agonist/antagonist agent, approved for the treatment of opioid dependence).[89,90] Advantages of buprenorphine may include a lower incidence of side effects (eg, sedation, respiratory depression) and fewer withdrawal symptoms on downward titration and discontinuation.

Some have designed protocols combining opioid antagonist and α_2 agonists for rapid detoxification.[91,92] Similarly, others have combined naltrexone and buprenorphine for short opioid detoxification protocol.[93] Recently, an ultrashort opioid

Table 1
Management of opioid intoxication

1. Discontinuation of all forms of opioid use (eg, surreptitious drug use, removal of transdermal delivery system)
2. There is no evidence that the use of activated charcoal or gastric lavage is of use, and may complicate treatment because of their own inherited side effects; similarly, hemodialysis is of little use
3. Obtain comprehensive toxicology screening to assess for the possibility of co-ingestion of other substances, including licit and over-the-counter substances (eg, alcohol, acetaminophen), illicit substances (eg, cocaine, (δ-9-tetrahydrocannabinol), and prescribed substances (eg, BZs, barbiturates, anticonvulsants)
4. Monitor vital signs (eg, respiratory rate, pulse oxymetry, blood gases, temperature), initiate supportive measures (eg, hydration and electrolyte replacement, oxygen supplementation), and maintain or establish an airway (eg, intubate if needed)
5. Assess and treat comorbid medical problems (eg, infections, head injury)
6. Administer an opioid antagonist (ie, naloxone); the initial dose depends on the patient's respiratory status, not the level of consciousness; monitor for the possibility of opioid withdrawal in opioid-habituated individuals
7. In intoxication with multiple substances, the use of agent-specific antidote should be considered (eg, BZ antagonists); in such cases, monitor for the possibility of substance-specific withdrawal syndrome

Respiratory Status	Initial Naloxone Dose[87]
Spontaneous breathing	0.05 mg intravenously, repeat every 2 to 3 min as needed, or titrate upwards until respiratory rate is ≥12 beats/min
Apneic patients	0.2–1 mg intravenously, repeat every 2 to 3 min as needed and titrate upwards until respiratory rate is ≥12 beats/min
Patients in cardiorespiratory arrest	2 mg and titrate upwards until respiratory rate is ≥12 beats/min
Notes:	1. If there has been no response after a total of 10 mg, reconsider diagnosis of opioid toxicity 2. Naloxone may be administered via intramuscular or subcutaneous routes, if intravenous route is unavailable 3. Repeated doses may be required at 1- to 2-h intervals depending on the type (ie, short- vs long-acting), amount, and time interval since the last administration of the narcotic

detoxification method has been introduced that requires patients to be anesthetized, intubated, and mechanically ventilated.[94,95] Patients are then given large bolus doses of naloxone, which precipitates acute opioid withdrawal while the patient is unconscious, and diuretics are administered to enhance opioid excretion.

The adjunct use of several substances may minimize withdrawal symptoms and facilitate opioid titration. Main among these is the use of α_2 adrenergic agonist agents (eg, clonidine, dexmedetomidine).[89,96,97] Similarly, muscle relaxant agents (eg, baclofen) and antidiarrheal agents (eg, diphenoxylate hydrochloride/atropine sulfate, loperamide hydrochloride) may be added for control of muscle spasms, aches, and gastrointestinal (GI) distress (**Box 6**).

Management of Opioid Dependence

The long-term management of opioid dependence is beyond the scope of this review and has been described in detail elsewhere.[98] Treatment seems to include one of 3

Table 2
Symptom of opioid withdrawal

Time from Last Use[a]	Withdrawal Symptoms
3–4 h after last use	Drug craving Anxiety Fear of withdrawal
8–14 h after last use	• Generalized malaise • Flu-like symptoms • Anxiety • Restlessness • Insomnia • Yawning • Rhinorrhea • Lacrimation • Diaphoresis • Abdominal cramps • Mydriasis
1–3 d after last use	• Tremor • Muscle spasms • GI distress: nausea, vomiting, diarrhea • Hypertension • Tachycardia • Hyperthermia • Chills • Piloerection

[a] The time to onset of opioid withdrawal symptoms depends on the half-life of the substance being used. This example assumes the use of a short-acting opioid (eg, heroin).

options: the use of long-acting opioid agents plus supportive therapy as in a methadone maintenance program; the use of opioid antagonist agent (ie, naltrexone); or the use of a partial opioid agonist agent (ie, buprenorphine).

BZS
Epidemiology

BZs are among the most commonly used prescribed substances in the world. According to the 2008 survey, there were 181,000 new sedatives users in the United States.[1] BZs are anxiolytics, hypnotics, amnesics, muscle relaxants, antiemetics, mood stabilizers, and anticonvulsants.[99] They are also the treatment of choice for the management of AWS,[25,27,28,45] akathisia,[100] and catatonia.[101]

Mechanism of Action

BZs have 2 main mechanisms of action: they have $GABA_A$-BZ subreceptors agonist activity, increasing the frequency of the chloride ion channel opening at the $GABA_A$ receptor, thus increasing the potency of GABA (different from barbiturates that are $GABA_A$ receptor agonists at the α subunit [increasing the duration of chloride ion channel opening at the $GABA_A$ receptor, thus increasing the potency of GABA]). BZs also inhibit acetylcholine release in basal forebrain and hippocampal synapses, which contributes to its sedative and amnesic effects.

All BZs act in a similar fashion. Yet, there are significant differences among them based on their molecular structure, onset of action, half-life, metabolism, and the presence of active metabolites (**Table 3; Fig. 5**).

| Box 6 |
| Management of opioid withdrawal |

Objective signs of withdrawal:

Pulse 10 beats/min > baseline, or *P*>90

SBP >10 mm Hg (above baseline), or blood pressure >160/95

Dilated pupils

Sweating, gooseflesh, rhinorrhea, lacrimation

Methadone:

Methadone 10 mg by mouth/intravenously should reverse most symptoms

First dose is administered when 2 of 4 symptoms are present (see objective signs of withdrawal)

Administer methadone 10 mg by mouth/intravenously every 4 hours as needed, × 24 hours

Rarely >40 mg are needed; but total dose depends on the patient's tolerance level

On day 2 the total methadone dose required on day 1 may be administered on a once-a-day or twice-a-day schedule, depending on the dose and practitioner's preference

Given the long half-life of methadone once-a-day dosing is sufficient

If the total dose is too large (eg, >60 mg/d) the dose may be divided to minimize side effects (eg, sedation, hypotension)

From day 3 on: the dose is tapered by 10%/d or 5 mg/d based on physician's preference and patient's tolerability

Buprenorphine:

A partial agonist/antagonist agent FDA-approved for the treatment of opioid dependence

Advantages of this agent may include a lower incidence of side effects (eg, sedation, respiratory depression) and fewer withdrawal symptoms on downward titration and discontinuation

Clonidine:

Clonidine, an α_2 agonist, may suppress or reverse symptoms of opioid withdrawal, and may be used alone or more commonly with methadone

Clonidine has no abuse potential

Dose: 0.1–0.3 mg/d (divided three times a day) administered either orally or transdermally

Hold dose if blood pressure decreases to less than 90/60 mm Hg

After stabilization for 14 days, taper dose over 4–6 days

Side effects include orthostatic hypotension, sedation, dry mouth, and constipation

For muscle cramps:

Baclofen 5 to 10 mg by mouth three times a day

For diarrhea and abdominal cramping:

Diphenoxylate hydrochloride/atropine sulfate (2 tablets four times a day, as needed, up to 20 mg/d), or

Loperamide hydrochloride (4 mg, followed by 2 mg after each loose stool up to a maximum of 16 mg/d)

Table 3
Pharmacologic characteristic of BZs

Generic Name	Trade Name	Class	Equipotency	Usual Daily Dose (mg)	Onset of Action[f]	Elimination Half-life (h)
Alprazolam	Xanax[a,b]	BZ	0.5	0.75–4	R	12–15
Clonazepam	Klonopin[a]	BZ	0.25	0.25–4	I	18–50
Lorazepam	Ativan[c,b]	BZ	1.0	0.5–6	I	10–15
Midazolam	Versed	BZ	2.5	Intravenous drip	UR	1–5
Diazepam	Valium	BZ	5.0	2–40	R	30–100[d]
Clorazepate	Tranxene	BZ	7.5	7.5–60	R	30–200[d]
Chlordiazepoxide	Librium	BZ	10	10–100	S	15–100[d]
Prazepam	Centrax	BZ	10	10–60	I	30–100[d]
Oxazepam	Serax[c]	BZ	15	15–60	S	3–15
Hypnotics						
Triazolam	Halcion[b]	BZ	2	0.125–0.5	R	2–4
Temazepam	Restoril	BZ	15	15–30	R	4–20
Flurazepam	Dalmane	BZ	15	15–30	R	47–100[d]
Estazolam	Prosom	BZ	2	1–2	R	10–24
Quazepam	Doral	BZ	?	7.5–15	R	25–40[d]
Zolpidem tartrate	Ambien[e]	Imidazopyridine, GABA$_{A1}$, Ω	?	10–20	R	1.4–2[d]
Zaleplon	Sonata[e]	GABA$_{A1}$, Ω	?	5–20	R	1[d]
Eszopiclone	Lunesta[e]	GABA$_{A1}$, Ω	?	2–3	R	5–6[d]

[a] Metabolized by alternative, nonoxidative pathways.
[b] Good sublingual absorption.
[c] Metabolized only by glucuronidation, usually unaffected by hepatic failure/all other required oxidative metabolism.
[d] Active metabolites are present.
[e] These agents lack the anxiolytic, muscle relaxant, and anticonvulsant effect of traditional BZs.
[f] Onset of action: I, intermediate; R, rapid; S, slow; UR, ultra rapid.

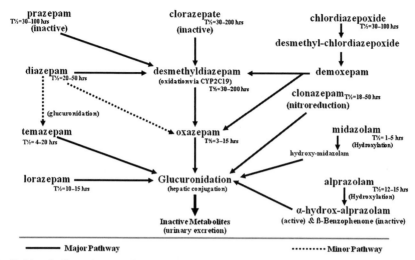

Fig. 5. Metabolic pathways of BZs.

BZ Intoxication

Diazepam and alprazolam are the 2 most widely abused BZs. Abusers often combine them with alcohol to enhance their effect. The concomitant use of BZs and alcohol or another CNS depressant is common in overdose. One of the advantages of BZs, compared with barbiturates, is their wide margin of safety (eg, they seldom produce coma or death), even at high doses, except when coadministered with other agents that may suppress respiratory drive (eg, alcohol, barbiturates, opioids). The signs and symptoms of BZ intoxication are, in general, a continuation of the primary BZ effect, namely anxiolysis and sedation. Thus, oversedation, slurred speech, ataxia, and depressed mental status are common, although infrequently there are cases of paradoxic inhibition and agitation. In extreme cases, particularly when another agent has been consumed, the consequence may be stupor, respiratory depression, and coma, or even death (**Table 4**).

Management of Acute Intoxication

When taken by themselves, BZs are seldom lethal, even when taken in an overdose.[102] In the hospital setting, as-needed administration is another source of BZ intoxication. It is particularly bad if the patient is receiving BZs parenterally, because intravenous BZs are diluted in propylene glycol (PG). Given its toxic effects, the prolonged administration of a BZ containing PG may lead to the development of hyperosmolality, hemolysis, skin and soft tissue necrosis (from extravasation), cardiac dysrhythmias, hypotension, lactic acidosis, seizure, coma, and multisystem organ failure.[103]

As in alcohol and opioid intoxication, the general treatment of BZ intoxication involves protection of airway, assessment of comorbid medical problems, discontinuation of the BZ and other CNS depressant agents, supportive measures (eg, respiratory rate, temperature, hydration), and the administration of a BZ antagonist (ie, flumazenil). Special attention is also required when there is a possibility of multiple drug intoxication (eg, suicidal overdose) because some substances, particularly CNS-depressant agents may potentiate the respiratory suppressant effect of BZs.

Flumazenil,[104] a BZ antagonist, is usually administered intravenously (initial dose 0.2 mg intravenously administered in 30 seconds), although it may be administered

Table 4
Characteristics of other substances of abuse

Class	Types	Classification	Common Names	Mechanism of Action	Signs of Acute Intoxication	Signs of Withdrawal

Stimulants	Caffeine	Xanthine alkaloid	Coffee	Nonselective antagonist of adenosine receptors	• Caffeine jitters
					• Usually >300 mg
					  Drowsiness
					  Restlessness
					  Nervousness
					  Irritability
					  Excitement
					  Insomnia
					  Facial flushing
					  Increased urination
					  Fasciculations
					  Circumstantiality
					  Tachycardia
					  Psychomotor agitation
						• Headache
						• Nausea
						• Crash
						  Drowsiness
						  Fatigue
						  Lack of motivation
						  Poor concentration
						  Irritability
						  Anxiety

	Nicotine	Natural liquid alkaloid	Cigarettes Cigars Smokeless tobacco Snuff Spit tobacco Bidis Chew	Nicotinic cholinergic receptor agonist	• GI distress: nausea, vomiting, diarrhea, abdominal cramps • Drooling • Headaches • Shortness of breath, dyspnea • Pallor • Sweating • Weakness • Incoordination • Palpitations • Cardiac arrhythmias • Seizures	• Cravings for nicotine • Irritability • Insomnia • Fatigue • Inability to concentrate • Headache • Cough • Sore throat • GI distress: constipation, flatulence, abdominal pain • Dry mouth • Postnasal drip • Tightness in the chest

Drug	Description	Street names	Mechanism	Intoxication	Withdrawal
Amphetamine Methamphetamine	Racemic β-phenyliso-propylamine; a phenylethylamine	Speed Meth Crank Chalk Ice Crystal Glass Fire	Exerts its effects by binding to the monoamine transporters and increasing extracellular levels of the biogenic amines DA, NE, $5\text{-}HT_3$	• Restlessness • Dizziness • Tremors • Chest pains • Hypertension • Talkativeness • Hyperactive reflexes • Insomnia • Euphoria • Psychosis • Confusion • Assaultiveness • Paranoia • Hallucinations • Suicidality • Homicidality	• Anxiety • Irritability • Agitation • Fatigue • Hypersomnolence • Depression • Increased appetite • Psychosis • Suicidality
MDMA (3,4-methylenedio-xymetham-phetamine)	Phenylethylamine: a psychedelic with LSD & amphetaminelike qualities	Ecstasy E Eve X XTC Adam Clarity Love drug Lovers' speed STP	Inhibits the vesicular monoamine transporter, leading to increased concentrations of $5\text{-}HT_3$, NE and DA; weak $5\text{-}HT_1$ and 5-HT receptor agonist	• Anxiety • Paranoia • Panic attacks • Myoclonus • Hyperreflexia • Shortness of breath, tachypnea • Palpitations • Cardiac arrhythmia • Hyperthermia • Hyponatremia • Seizures • Hypervigilance • Derealization • Hallucinations • Delusions • Thought disorder • Disorientation • Confusion • Cognitive impairment • Memory impairment • Delirium	No withdrawal state has been described

(continued on next page)

Table 4
(*continued*)

Class	Types	Classification	Common Names	Mechanism of Action	Signs of Acute Intoxication	Signs of Withdrawal
	Cocaine	Benzoylmethy-legonine (ecgonine is an amino alcohol base closely related to tropine, the amino alcohol in atropine)	Coke Crack Snow Flake Blow	$5\text{-}HT_3$, NE and DA reuptake inhibitor → enhancing monoamino transmission	• Alertness • Feelings of well-being • Euphoria • Increased energy and motor activity • Feelings of competence and sexuality • Followed by: Anxiety Paranoia Restlessness • With excessive dosage: Tremors Convulsions Hyperthermia • Dose-dependent, end-organ toxicity in virtually every organ system in the body, primarily through hemody-namic effects	• Crash: Depression Anxiety Fatigue Difficulty concentrating Anhedonia Increased cocaine craving Increased appetite Increased sleep Increased dreaming (because of increased rapid-eye movement sleep)

Hallucinogens					
Lysergic acid diethylamide (LSD)	Psychedelic	5-HT$_{2A}$ receptor binding	Acid Blotter Dots Boomers Cubes Microdot Yellow sunshine	• General effects: Dizziness Weakness Drowsiness Nausea Hyperthermia Euphoria Expansiveness Depersonalization Paresthesias Synesthesias Feeling of inner tension relieved by laughing or crying Time distortion Visual illusions (micropsia, wavelike perceptions) • High doses: Dysphoria An overwhelming sense of dread Panic reactions Disorientation Hallucinations • Cardiovascular collapse with large ingestions, >400 µg	No withdrawal state has been described No withdrawal state has been described

(continued on next page)

Table 4
(continued)

Class	Types	Classification	Common Names	Mechanism of Action	Signs of Acute Intoxication	Signs of Withdrawal

	Phencyclidine (PCP)	A dissociative anesthetic with pharmacologic properties similar to ketamine	Angel dust
			Ozone
			Wack
			Rocket fuel
			Boat
			Hog
			Peace pill
				Non-competitive antagonist of N-methyl-D-aspartate (NMDA) receptors	• Low doses:
					  Social withdrawal
					  Dissociation
					  Visual and auditory distortion
					• High doses:
					  Disorientation
					  Severe agitation
					  Violent behavior
					  Auditory hallucinations
					  Catatonic stupor
					  Bizarre or violent behavior
					  Nystagmus (vertical and horizontal)
					  Incoordination
					  Coma
						No withdrawal state has been described

	Mescaline (3,4,5-trimethoxy-phenethylamine)	Psychedelic alkaloid of the phenylethylamine class	Peyote Buttons Cactus Mesc	5-HT$_{2A}$ receptor binding, partial agonist	Produce neuropsychiatric effects similar to LSD Nausea and vomiting frequently precede the onset of psychedelic effects	No withdrawal state has been described

					No withdrawal state has been described
	Psilocybin	Psychedelic indole of the tryptamine family	Mushroom Magic mushrooms Sacred mushrooms Shrooms Purple passion	5-HT$_{1A}$ and 5-HT$_{2A}$ receptor binding, partial agonist	Produce neuropsychiatric effects similar to LSD
Cannabinoids	THC (δ-9-tetrahydro-cannabinol) Hashish	Cannabinoids	Marijuana Weed Dope Grass Herb Joint Pot Reefer Mary Jane Marihuana Boom Chronic Gangster Hash Hash oil Hemp	Cannabinoid (CB$_1$ and CB$_2$) receptor agonists leading to activation of multiple intracellular signal transduction pathways	• Euphoria • Slowed thinking and reaction time • Confusion • Impaired balance and coordination • Cough • Frequent respiratory infections • Impaired memory and learning • Increased heart rate • Anxiety • Panic attacks	• Marijuana craving • Negative mood (eg, feeling miserable) • Irritability • Anxiety • Muscle pain • Chills • Decreased food intake • Insomnia

(continued on next page)

Table 4
(continued)

Class	Types	Classification	Common Names	Mechanism of Action	Signs of Acute Intoxication	Signs of Withdrawal
CNS Depressants	Barbiturates BZs		Amytal Nembutal Seconal Phenobarbital Barbs Reds Red birds Phennies Tooies Yellows Yellow jackets Ativan Halcion Librium Valium Xanax Candy Downers Sleeping pills Tranks	$GABA_A$ receptor agonist at the α subunit (increasing the duration of chloride ion channel opening at the $GABA_A$ receptor [increasing the potency of GABA]) AMPA receptor antagonist (type of GLU receptor) $GABA_A$-BZ subreceptors agonist (increasing the frequency of the chloride ion channel opening at the $GABA_A$ receptor [increasing the potency of GABA]) Inhibits acetylcholine release in basal forebrain and hippocampal Synapses	• Reduced anxiety • Feeling of well-being • Lowered inhibitions • Slowed pulse and breathing • Lowered blood pressure • Sedation • Drowsiness • Dizziness • Poor concentration • Fatigue • Depression • Confusion • Impaired coordination • Slurred speech • Impaired memory • Impaired judgment • Respiratory depression and arrest • Death	Common: • Insomnia • GI distress • Tremors • Agitation • Fearfulness • Muscle spasms Less Common: • Irritability • Diaphoresis • Depersonalization • Derealization • Hypersensitivity to stimuli • Depression • Suicidal ideation Life-threatening withdrawal: • Psychosis • Seizures • Catatonia • DTs

γ-Hydroxybutyric acid (GHB)	γ-Hydroxybutyrate G Georgia home boy Grievous bodily harm Liquid ecstasy Date rape drug	GHB receptor agonist Weak agonist at the GABA$_B$ receptor Its effect on DA release is biphasic: low concentrations stimulate DA release via the GHB receptor; Higher concentrations inhibit DA release via GABA$_B$ receptors	• Drowsiness • Nausea/vomiting • Headache • Loss of consciousness • Loss of reflexes • Seizures • Coma • Death	• Anxiety • Restlessness • Insomnia • Tremor • Tachycardia • Hypertension • Diaphoresis • Hyperthermia • GI distress • Anorexia • Nightmares • Agitation • Hallucinations • Delirium

by mouth.[104] It has a short half-life (0.7–1.0 hours), thus depending on the half-life of the BZ being treated, it may require repeated drug administration (at 20-minute intervals) or the use of a continuous drip, for a maximum dose of 3 mg/h.[104] Flumazenil may trigger BZ withdrawal in habituated individuals (**Table 5**).[105]

Table 5
Management of BZ intoxication

1. Discontinuation all BZ and other CNS-depressant use
2. There is no evidence that the administration of activated charcoal or gastric lavage is of use, and they may complicate treatment because of their own inherited side effects. Similarly, hemodialysis is of little use
3. Obtain comprehensive toxicology screening to assess for the possibility of co-ingestion of other substances, including licit (eg, ethanol) and over-the-counter substances (eg, alcohol, acetaminophen), illicit substances (eg, cocaine, THC), and prescribed substances (eg, opioids, barbiturates, anticonvulsants)
4. Monitor vital signs (eg, respiratory rate, pulse oxymetry, blood gases, temperature) and electrocardiography.
5. Initiate supportive measures (eg, hydration and electrolyte replacement, oxygen supplementation)
6. Maintain or establish an airway (eg, intubate if needed)
7. Assess and treat comorbid medical problems (eg, infections, head injury)
8. Administer BZ antagonist, flumazenil,[104] as indicated in the following chart
   - The peak effect of a single flumazenil dose occurs approximately 6 to 10 minutes after intravenous administration
   - The duration of flumazenil is short (0.7–1.3 hours); thus, the duration of effect of a long-acting BZ or a large BZ dose can exceed that of flumazenil
   - Monitor for the possibility of BZ withdrawal in the case of BZ-habituated individuals
   - Because oral BZ overdose has a low rate of morbidity and mortality is rare, the risks of flumazenil treatment often outweigh its benefits
9. In intoxication with multiple substances the use of agent-specific antidote should be considered (eg, opioid antagonists); monitor for the possibility of substance specific withdrawal syndrome

Stage	Flumazenil Dose[87]
Initial dose	0.2 mg intravenously over 30 s; if desired level of consciousness not obtained after an additional 30 s: an additional dose of 0.3 mg intravenously may be given over 30 s
Repeat doses	Further doses of 0.5 mg intravenously over 30 s may be given at 1-min intervals, if needed, to maximum total dose of 3 mg
Maximum total cumulative dose	Patients with only partial response after 3 mg may require additional slow titration (as mentioned earlier) to a total dose of 5 mg If no response 5 min after receiving total dose of 5 mg, overdose is unlikely to be BZ and further treatment with flumazenil will likely not help
Resedation	After intoxication with high doses of BZs, the duration of a single dose of flumazenil is not expected to exceed 1 h; if desired, the period of wakefulness may be prolonged with repeated low intravenous doses of flumazenil (ie, repeated doses may be given at 20-min intervals if needed; for repeat treatment, no more than 1 mg [given as 0.5 mg/min] should be given at any one time and no more than 3 mg should be given in any 1 h), or by an infusion of 0.1–0.4 mg/h

Management of BZ Withdrawal

All substances that enhance GABA activity are associated with the development of tolerance and withdrawal syndromes (including autonomic hyperactivity, agitation, irritability, craving, confusion, delirium, and seizures). Several cases of catatonia induced by or associated with BZ withdrawal have been reported.[106]

As with other CNS-depressant agents (eg, alcohol, barbiturates) withdrawal symptoms may begin in the presence of relative (eg, decreased dose or change in formulation from long to short half-life) or absolute abstinence from BZs. Therefore, withdrawal symptom may be triggered by changes in regimen (eg, dosing, formulation), noncompliance with medication taking, or other psychosocial factors (eg, running out of medication, the patient deciding they do not need it any longer, not liking side effects).

As detailed in **Table 4**, the signs and symptoms of BZ withdrawal are similar to those of AWS (eg, tremors, diaphoresis, insomnia, anxiety, irritability, agitation), and are potentially life-threatening (eg, confusion, psychosis, catatonia, seizures, death). The onset of the symptoms reflects the pharmacokinetics of the substance one is habituated to (ie, the half-life of BZ) and the specifics of the pattern of abuse (eg, frequency of use, total daily dose, rate of decrease, use of other concomitant CNS depressants).

As in other CNS depressants, treatment of withdrawal symptoms usually requires the reintroduction of the offending agent and a slow, controlled taper. The use of long-acting (eg, chlordiazepoxide, diazepam) agents is preferred, because the long-acting metabolites are expected to provide a smooth titration and minimize withdrawal symptoms on tapering.

The use of a BZ to manage the long-term problem of BZ abuse and dependence, although effective in preventing withdrawal syndromes, seems counterproductive and, to some, it just perpetuates the problem. Others have reported on the successful use of other GABA-ergic agents as substitutes for BZs. There are reports on the use of carbamazepine,[107] valproate,[108] gabapentin,[109] topiramate,[110] and oxcarbazepine.[111]

Management of BZ Dependence

The long-term management of BZ dependence is beyond the scope of this review and has been described in detail elsewhere.[112–114] In general, conversion to a long-acting agent and a slow taper over time have been the treatment of choice, coupled with appropriate pharmacologic management of comorbid psychiatric symptoms (eg, management of underlying anxiety disorder) or other coexisting substance abuse problem (eg, alcohol abuse). In addition, psychotherapeutic approaches may help patients cope better with the transition off substances.

NICOTINE
Epidemiology

The 2008 NSDAH survey found that 70.9 million Americans (or 28.4%) of the population aged 12 years or older were current (past month) users of a tobacco product.[1] Males (compared with females) had higher rates of use of each specific tobacco product: cigarettes (26.3 vs 21.7%), cigars (9.0 vs 1.7%), smokeless tobacco (6.8 vs 0.4%), and pipe tobacco (1.2 vs 0.3%). The prevalence of current use of a tobacco product varied widely depending on race or ethnicity. It was greater for American Indians or Alaska Natives (48.7%) and lowest among Asians (13.9%), with Hispanics (21.3%), blacks (28.6%), and whites (30.4%) in between. The use of illicit drugs and alcohol was more common among current cigarette smokers than among nonsmokers.

Mechanism of Action

Nicotine is a liquid alkaloid found in tobacco and other plants. Once ingested, nicotine is readily absorbed, quickly distributed, and easily crosses the brain-blood barrier. It has a short half-life (2 hours) and it undergoes hepatic metabolism via the cytochrome P450 system (CYP2A6 and CYP2B6). Nicotine is an acetylcholine receptor agonist that seems to trigger several neurochemical events, including the release of NE and DA; the release of growth hormone, cortisol, antiduretic hormone, and glycerol; and depending on the dose, it increases or decreases the release of acetylcholine. By stimulating the chemoreceptor trigger zone it causes nausea and vomiting.

Nicotine Intoxication

Although not common, patients can present with signs of nicotine intoxication (GI distress [eg, nausea, salivation, abdominal pain, vomiting, diarrhea]; CNS symptoms [eg, headache, dizziness, hearing and visual disturbance, confusion, weakness, exhaustion, lack of coordination, seizures]; and cardiac complaints [eg, chest pain, shortness of breath, arrhythmias]), associated with the concomitant use of tobacco products and nicotine replacement delivery systems.

Management of Nicotine Withdrawal

In general, the acute management of nicotine withdrawal includes the use of a nicotine replacement therapy (NRT) system and slow titration (see later discussion).

Management of Nicotine Dependence

The long-term management of nicotine dependence is beyond the scope of this review and has been described in detail elsewhere.[115–117] In general, there are several treatment options, including NRT (which includes gum, lozenges, transdermal patch, inhaler, and nasal spray delivery systems, which all provide nicotine to a smoker without using tobacco). The idea is to relieve patients from nicotine withdrawal symptoms as they work the habit. In general, NRTs increase the rate of quitting by 50% to 70%.[118] Their success increases when combined with hypnosis or a counseling program.[119] Varenicline (a nicotine receptor partial agonist)[120] had a continuous quit rate for any 4 weeks of 48% (dose 1.0 mg twice daily) compared with 33% on bupropion and 17% for placebo.[121] Bupropion (a DA/NE reuptake inhibitor) has shown a smoking cessation success rate of 44% (vs placebo 19%).[122] Some have shown an added benefit of combining bupropion and varenicline.[123] In selected, highly suggestible patients hypnosis has shown excellent results, with up to 81% to 90% success rates.[124] There are also various psychotherapeutic techniques, including CBT,[125] group therapy,[126] motivational advice by clinicians,[127] and motivational interviewing.[128]

OTHER SUBSTANCES OF ABUSE

Other substances of abuse include psychostimulants, anticholinergic effects, and hallucinogens. A full description of the mechanisms of action, effects, and management of these substances is beyond the scope of this review, but **Table 4** summarizes the essentials for their recognition and acute management by general practitioners. None of these agents has a specific antidote. Treatment of the acute intoxication is usually supportive, with various pharmacologic agents used for symptomatic management.

It is possible to obtain emergent consultation with a medical toxicologist by calling the United States Poison Control Network at 1 800 222 1222, or access the World

Health Organization's list of international poison centers (http://www.who.int/ipcs/poisons/centre/directory/en).

REFERENCES

1. SAMHSA. Results from the 2008 national survey on drug use and health: national findings. Rockville (MD): Substance Abuse and Mental Health Services Administration (SAMHSA); 2009.
2. DHHS. Acamprosate: a new medication for alcohol use disorders. 2009. Available at: www.kap.samhsa.gov/products/brochures/advisory/text/Acamprosate-Advisory.doc. Accessed July 29, 2009.
3. Schellhorn SE, Barnhill JW, Raiteri V, et al. A comparison of psychiatric consultation between geriatric and non-geriatric medical inpatients. Int J Geriatr Psychiatry 2009;24(10):1054–61.
4. Williams GD, Stinson FS, Lane JD, et al. Apparent per capita alcohol consumption: national, state and regional trends, 1977–94. Bethesda (MD): NloAAa, Alcoholism;1996. p. 3–6.
5. Lieber CS. Medical disorders of alcoholism. N Engl J Med 1995;333(16): 1058–65.
6. Robins LN, Helzer JE, Weissman MM, et al. Lifetime prevalence of specific psychiatric disorders in three sites. Arch Gen Psychiatry 1984;41(10):949–58.
7. Mokdad AH, Marks JS, Stroup DF, et al. Actual causes of death in the United States, 2000 [see comment]. JAMA 2004;291(10):1238–45 [erratum appears in JAMA 2005;293(3):293–4; PMID: 15657315].
8. Moore RD, Bone LR, Geller G, et al. Prevalence, detection, and treatment of alcoholism in hospitalized patients. JAMA 1989;261(3):403–7.
9. Kennedy WJ. Chemical dependency: a treatable disease. Ohio State Med J 1985;81(2):77–9.
10. Saitz R, Friedman LS, Mayo-Smith MF. Alcohol withdrawal: a nationwide survey of inpatient treatment practices. J Gen Intern Med 1995;10(9):479–87.
11. Faingold CL, N'Gouemo P, Riaz A. Ethanol and neurotransmitter interactions–from molecular to integrative effects. Prog Neurobiol 1998;55(5):509–35.
12. Tsai G, Coyle JT. The role of glutamatergic neurotransmission in the pathophysiology of alcoholism. Annu Rev Med 1998;49:173–84.
13. Di Chiara G, Imperato A. Preferential stimulation of dopamine release in the nucleus accumbens by opiates, alcohol, and barbiturates: studies with transcerebral dialysis in freely moving rats. Ann N Y Acad Sci 1986;473:367–81.
14. Cagetti E, Liang J, Spigelman I, et al. Withdrawal from chronic intermittent ethanol treatment changes subunit composition, reduces synaptic function, and decreases behavioral responses to positive allosteric modulators of GABAA receptors. Mol Pharmacol 2003;63(1):53–64.
15. Hawley RJ, Nemeroff CB, Bissette G, et al. Neurochemical correlates of sympathetic activation during severe alcohol withdrawal. Alcohol Clin Exp Res 1994; 18(6):1312–6.
16. Sjoquist B, Perdahl E, Winblad B. The effect of alcoholism on salsolinol and biogenic amines in human brain. Drug Alcohol Depend 1983;12(1):15–23.
17. Pohorecky LA. Influence of alcohol on peripheral neurotransmitter function. Fed Proc 1982;41(8):2452–5.
18. Perec CJ, Celener D, Tiscornia OM, et al. Effects of chronic ethanol administration on the autonomic innervation of salivary glands, pancreas and heart. Am J Gastroenterol 1979;72(1):46–59.

19. Linnoila M, Mefford I, Nutt D, et al. NIH conference. Alcohol withdrawal and noradrenergic function. Ann Intern Med 1987;107(6):875–89.
20. Gonzales R, Bungay PM, Kilanmaa K, et al. In vivo links between neurochemistry and behavioral effects of ethanol. Alcohol Clin Exp Res 1996;20(Suppl 8): 203A–9A.
21. Nakamura J, Uchimura N, Yamada S, et al. Does plasma free-3-methoxy-4-hydroxyphenyl(ethylene)glycol increase in the delirious state? A comparison of the effects of mianserin and haloperidol on delirium. Int Clin Psychopharmacol 1997;12(3):147–52.
22. Maldonado JR. Pathoetiological model of delirium: a comprehensive understanding of the neurobiology of delirium and an evidence-based approach to prevention and treatment. Crit Care Clin 2008;24(4):789–856.
23. Esel E. [Neurobiology of alcohol withdrawal inhibitory and excitatory neurotransmitters]. Turk Psikiyatri Derg 2006;17(2):129–37 [in Turkish].
24. Holbrook AM, Crowther R, Lotter A, et al. Meta-analysis of benzodiazepine use in the treatment of acute alcohol withdrawal. CMAJ 1999;160(5):649–55.
25. Maldonado JR, Brooks JO, Nguyen LH, et al. A comparison of lorazepam versus diazepam in the treatment of alcohol withdrawal, Submitted, 2010.
26. Maldonado JR, DiMartini A, Owen J. Psychopharmacological treatment of substance use disorders in the medically ill. In: Ferrando S, Levenson J, Robinson M, et al, editors. Clinical handbook of psychopharmacology in the medically ill. Arlington (VA): American Psychiatric Publishing; 2010. p. 537–55.
27. Mayo-Smith MF, Beecher LH, Fischer TL, et al. Management of alcohol withdrawal delirium. An evidence-based practice guideline. Arch Intern Med 2004;164(13):1405–12.
28. Ntais C, Pakos E, Kyzas P, et al. Benzodiazepines for alcohol withdrawal. Cochrane Database Syst Rev 2005;3:CD005063.
29. Sullivan JT, Sykora K, Schneiderman J, et al. Assessment of alcohol withdrawal: the revised clinical institute withdrawal assessment for alcohol scale (CIWA-Ar). Br J Addict 1989;84(11):1353–7.
30. Wetterling T, Kanitz RD, Besters B, et al. A new rating scale for the assessment of the alcohol-withdrawal syndrome (AWS scale). Alcohol Alcohol 1997;32(6): 753–60.
31. Kosten TR, O'Connor PG. Management of drug and alcohol withdrawal. N Engl J Med 2003;348(18):1786–95.
32. Kuhr BM. Prolonged delirium with propanolol. J Clin Psychiatry 1979;40(4): 198–9.
33. Rathlev NK, Medzon R, Lowery D, et al. Intracranial pathology in elders with blunt head trauma. Acad Emerg Med 2006;13(3):302–7.
34. Malcolm R, Myrick H, Roberts J, et al. The effects of carbamazepine and lorazepam on single versus multiple previous alcohol withdrawals in an outpatient randomized trial. J Gen Intern Med 2002;17(5):349–55.
35. Stuppaeck CH, Pycha R, Miller C, et al. Carbamazepine versus oxazepam in the treatment of alcohol withdrawal: a double-blind study. Alcohol Alcohol 1992; 27(2):153–8.
36. Polycarpou A, Papanikolaou P, Ioannidis JP, et al. Anticonvulsants for alcohol withdrawal. Cochrane Database Syst Rev 2005;3:CD005064.
37. Schik G, Wedegaertner FR, Liersch J, et al. Oxcarbazepine versus carbamazepine in the treatment of alcohol withdrawal. Addict Biol 2005;10(3): 283–8.

38. Croissant B, Diehl A, Klein O, et al. A pilot study of oxcarbazepine versus acamprosate in alcohol-dependent patients. Alcohol Clin Exp Res 2006; 30(4):630–5.
39. Krupitsky EM, Rudenko AA, Burakov AM, et al. Antiglutamatergic strategies for ethanol detoxification: comparison with placebo and diazepam. Alcohol Clin Exp Res 2007;31(4):604–11.
40. Myrick H, Malcolm R, Randall PK, et al. A double-blind trial of gabapentin versus lorazepam in the treatment of alcohol withdrawal. Alcohol Clin Exp Res 2009; 33(9):1582–8.
41. Becker HC, Myrick H, Veatch LM. Pregabalin is effective against behavioral and electrographic seizures during alcohol withdrawal. Alcohol Alcohol 2006;41(4): 399–406.
42. Martinotti G, di Nicola M, Frustaci A, et al. Pregabalin, tiapride and lorazepam in alcohol withdrawal syndrome: a multi-centre, randomized, single-blind comparison trial. Addiction 2010;105(2):288–99.
43. Myrick H, Taylor B, LaRowe S, et al. A retrospective chart review comparing tiagabine and benzodiazepines for the treatment of alcohol withdrawal. J Psychoactive Drugs 2005;37(4):409–14.
44. Stuppaeck CH, Deisenhammer EA, Kurz M, et al. The irreversible gamma-aminobutyrate transaminase inhibitor vigabatrin in the treatment of the alcohol withdrawal syndrome. Alcohol Alcohol 1996;31(1):109–11.
45. Stern TA, Gross AF, Stern TW, et al. Current approaches to the recognition and treatment of alcohol withdrawal and delirium tremens. Prim Care Companion J Clin Psychiatry 2010;12(3):e1–9.
46. Baumgartner GR, Rowen RC. Transdermal clonidine versus chlordiazepoxide in alcohol withdrawal: a randomized, controlled clinical trial. South Med J 1991; 84(3):312–21.
47. Dobrydnjov I, Axelsson K, Berggren L, et al. Intrathecal and oral clonidine as prophylaxis for postoperative alcohol withdrawal syndrome: a randomized double-blinded study. Anesth Analg 2004;98(3):738–44.
48. Riihioja P, et al. Effects of dexmedetomidine on rat locus coeruleus and ethanol withdrawal symptoms during intermittent ethanol exposure. Alcohol Clin Exp Res 1999;23(3):432–8.
49. Cooper L, et al. Adjuvant use of dexmedetomidine may reduce the incidence of endotracheal intubation caused by benzodiazepines in the treatment of delirium tremens. Presented at the 2005 annual meeting of the American Society of Anesthesiology. Anesthesiology 2005;103:A31–7.
50. Kandiah P, Jacob S, Pandya D, et al. Novel use of dexmedetomidine in 7 adults with resistant alcohol withdrawal in the ICU. Presented at the 2009 annual meeting of the Society of Critical Care Medicine 2009.
51. Rovasalo A, Tohmo H, Aantaa R, et al. Dexmedetomidine as an adjuvant in the treatment of alcohol withdrawal delirium: a case report. Gen Hosp Psychiatry 2006;28(4):362–3.
52. Marcantonio ER, Juarez G, Goldman L, et al. The relationship of postoperative delirium with psychoactive medications. JAMA 1994;272(19):1518–22.
53. Maldonado JR. Delirium in the acute care setting: characteristics, diagnosis and treatment. Crit Care Clin 2008;24(4):657–722, vii.
54. Pandharipande P, Shintani A, Peterson J, et al. Lorazepam is an independent risk factor for transitioning to delirium in intensive care unit patients. Anesthesiology 2006;104(1):21–6.

55. Tune LE, Bylsma FW. Benzodiazepine-induced and anticholinergic-induced delirium in the elderly. Int Psychogeriatr 1991;3(2):397–408.

56. Maldonado JR, Wysong A, van der Starre PJ, et al. Dexmedetomidine and the reduction of postoperative delirium after cardiac surgery. Psychosomatics 2009;50(3):206–17.

57. Garbutt JC. The state of pharmacotherapy for the treatment of alcohol dependence. J Subst Abuse Treat 2009;36(1):S15–23 [quiz: S24–5].

58. Hanwella R, de Silva V. Treatment of alcohol dependence. Ceylon Med J 2009; 54(2):63–5.

59. Swift RM. Drug therapy for alcohol dependence. N Engl J Med 1999;340(19): 1482–90.

60. Romo L. [Behavior and cognitive therapy for alcohol related disorders]. Soins Psychiatr 2008;257:26–8 [in French].

61. Carroll KM, Ball SA, Nich C, et al. Motivational interviewing to improve treatment engagement and outcome in individuals seeking treatment for substance abuse: a multisite effectiveness study. Drug Alcohol Depend 2006;81(3): 301–12.

62. Tariq L, van den Berg M, Hoogenveen RT, et al. Cost-effectiveness of an opportunistic screening programme and brief intervention for excessive alcohol use in primary care. PLoS One 2009;4(5):e5696.

63. Anton RF, Moak DH, Latham P, et al. Naltrexone combined with either cognitive behavioral or motivational enhancement therapy for alcohol dependence. J Clin Psychopharmacol 2005;25(4):349–57.

64. Feeney GF, Connor JP, Young RM, et al. Combined acamprosate and naltrexone, with cognitive behavioural therapy is superior to either medication alone for alcohol abstinence: a single centre's experience with pharmacotherapy. Alcohol Alcohol 2006;41(3):321–7.

65. Ferri M, Amato L, Davoli M. Alcoholics Anonymous and other 12-step programmes for alcohol dependence. Cochrane Database Syst Rev 2006;3: CD005032.

66. Raby K. Investigations on the disulfiram-alcohol reaction; clinical observations. Q J Stud Alcohol 1953;14(4):545–56.

67. de Sousa A. An open randomized study comparing disulfiram and acamprosate in the treatment of alcohol dependence. Alcohol Alcohol 2005;40(6): 545–8.

68. De Sousa A. A one-year pragmatic trial of naltrexone vs disulfiram in the treatment of alcohol dependence. Alcohol Alcohol 2004;39(6):528–31.

69. Malcolm R, Olive MF, Lechner W. The safety of disulfiram for the treatment of alcohol and cocaine dependence in randomized clinical trials: guidance for clinical practice. Expert Opin Drug Saf 2008;7(4):459–72.

70. Campral (Acamprosate Calcium) Home Page. 2010. Available at: http://www.prempharm.ca/Campral%20Product%20Monographs%20English.pdf. Accessed February 13, 2010.

71. Littleton J. Acamprosate in alcohol dependence: how does it work? Addiction 1995;90(9):1179–88.

72. Snyder JL, Bowers TG. The efficacy of acamprosate and naltrexone in the treatment of alcohol dependence: a relative benefits analysis of randomized controlled trials. Am J Drug Alcohol Abuse 2008;34(4):449–61.

73. Chick J, Anton R, Checinski K, et al. A multicentre, randomized, double-blind, placebo-controlled trial of naltrexone in the treatment of alcohol dependence or abuse. Alcohol Alcohol 2000;35(6):587–93.

74. De Sousa AA, De Sousa J, Kapoor H. An open randomized trial comparing disulfiram and topiramate in the treatment of alcohol dependence. J Subst Abuse Treat 2008;34(4):460–3.
75. Rubio G, Martinez-Gras I, Manzanares J. Modulation of impulsivity by topiramate: implications for the treatment of alcohol dependence. J Clin Psychopharmacol 2009;29(6):584–9.
76. Mason BJ, Light JM, Williams LD, et al. Proof-of-concept human laboratory study for protracted abstinence in alcohol dependence: effects of gabapentin. Addict Biol 2009;14(1):73–83.
77. Martinotti G, Di Nicola M, Tedeschi D, et al. Pregabalin versus naltrexone in alcohol dependence: a randomised, double-blind, comparison trial. J Psychopharmacol 2010;24:1367–74.
78. Addolorato G, Leggio L, Abenavoli L, et al. Baclofen in the treatment of alcohol withdrawal syndrome: a comparative study vs diazepam. Am J Med 2006; 119(3):276, e13–8.
79. Saitz R. Baclofen for alcohol withdrawal: not comparable to the gold standard (benzodiazepines). Am J Med 2007;120(6):e9 [author reply: e11].
80. Myrick H, Anton RF, Li X, et al. Effect of naltrexone and ondansetron on alcohol cue-induced activation of the ventral striatum in alcohol-dependent people. Arch Gen Psychiatry 2008;65(4):466–75.
81. Johnson BA, Ait-Daoud N, Ma JZ, et al. Ondansetron reduces mood disturbance among biologically predisposed, alcohol-dependent individuals. Alcohol Clin Exp Res 2003;27(11):1773–9.
82. Wang J, Christo PJ. The influence of prescription monitoring programs on chronic pain management. Pain Physician 2009;12(3):507–15.
83. NIDA. The brain & the actions of cocaine, opiates, and marijuana. The science of drug abuse & addiction 2009 [cited 2010 March 2010]; Available at: http://www.drugabuse.gov/pubs/teaching/Teaching4.html. Accessed July 27, 2009.
84. Zheng W. Activation of mu opioid receptor inhibits the excitatory glutamatergic transmission in the anterior cingulate cortex of the rats with peripheral inflammation. Eur J Pharmacol 2010;628(1–3):91–5.
85. Naloxone hydrochloride. In: MICROMEDEX® 1.0 [internet database] 2010, Thompson Reuters (Healthcare). Accessed March 14, 2010.
86. Dhalla IA, Mamdani MM, Sivilotti ML, et al. Prescribing of opioid analgesics and related mortality before and after the introduction of long-acting oxycodone. CMAJ 2009;181(12):891–6.
87. O'Connor PG, Kosten TR, Stine SM. Management of opioid intoxication and withdrawal. In: Graham AW, Schultz TK, Mayo-Smith MF, et al, editors. Principles of addiction medicine. Chevy Chase (MD): American Society of Addiction Medicine; 2003. p. 651–68.
88. Federal Register, Methadone: rules and regulations. Federal Register, 1989;54:8954.
89. Gowing L, Ali R, White J. Opioid antagonists and adrenergic agonists for the management of opioid withdrawal [update in Cochrane Database Syst Rev 2002;2:CD002021; PMID: 12076431]. Cochrane Database Syst Rev 2000;2:CD002021.
90. Gowing L, Ali R, White J. Buprenorphine for the management of opioid withdrawal [update of Cochrane Database Syst Rev 2004;4:CD002025; PMID: 15495026]. Cochrane Database Syst Rev 2006;2:CD002025.
91. Riordan CE, Kleber HD. Rapid opiate detoxification with clonidine and naloxone. Lancet 1980;1(8177):1079–80.

92. Vining E, Kosten TR, Kleber HD. Clinical utility of rapid clonidine-naltrexone detoxification for opioid abusers. Br J Addict 1988;83(5):567–75.

93. Umbricht A, Montoya ID, Hoover DR, et al. Naltrexone shortened opioid detoxification with buprenorphine. Drug Alcohol Depend 1999;56(3):181–90.

94. Albanese AP, Gevirtz C, Oppenheim B, et al. Outcome and six month follow up of patients after ultra rapid opiate detoxification (UROD). J Addict Dis 2000; 19(2):11–28.

95. O'Connor PG, Kosten TR. Rapid and ultrarapid opioid detoxification techniques [see comment]. JAMA 1998;279(3):229–34.

96. Finkel JC, Elrefai A. The use of dexmedetomidine to facilitate opioid and benzodiazepine detoxification in an infant. Anesth Analg 2004;98(6):1658–9.

97. Gold M, Redmond DE, Kleber HD. Clonidine blocks acute opiate withdrawal symptoms. Lancet 1978;2:599–600.

98. NIH Consensus Panel. NIH consensus panel recommends expanding access to and improving methadone treatment programs for heroin addiction. Eur Addict Res 1999;5:50–1.

99. Charney DS, Minic SJ, Harris RA. Hypnotics and sedatives. In: Hardman JG, Limbird LE, editors. Goodman and Gilman's: the pharmacological basis of therapeutics. 10th edition. New York: McGraw-Hill; 2001. p. 399–427.

100. Lima AR, Soares-Weiser K, Bacaltchuk J, et al. Benzodiazepines for neuroleptic-induced acute akathisia. Cochrane Database Syst Rev 2002;1:CD001950.

101. Greenfeld D, Conrad C, Kincare P, et al. Treatment of catatonia with low-dose lorazepam. Am J Psychiatry 1987;144(9):1224–5.

102. Hojer J, Baehrendtz S, Gustafsson L. Benzodiazepine poisoning: experience of 702 admissions to an intensive care unit during a 14-year period. J Intern Med 1989;226(2):117–22.

103. Wilson KC, Reardon C, Theodore AC, et al. Propylene glycol toxicity: a severe iatrogenic illness in ICU patients receiving IV benzodiazepines: a case series and prospective, observational pilot study. Chest 2005;128(3):1674–81.

104. Romazicon (Flumazenil) Home Page. 2009. Available at: www.rocheusa.com/products/romazicon/pi.pdf. Accessed July 29, 2009.

105. Weinbroum AA, Flaishon R, Sorkine P, et al. A risk-benefit assessment of flumazenil in the management of benzodiazepine overdose. Drug Saf 1997;17(3): 181–96.

106. Deuschle M, Lederbogen F. Benzodiazepine withdrawal-induced catatonia. Pharmacopsychiatry 2001;34(1):41–2.

107. Schweizer E, Rickels K, Case WG, et al. Carbamazepine treatment in patients discontinuing long-term benzodiazepine therapy. Effects on withdrawal severity and outcome. Arch Gen Psychiatry 1991;48(5):448–52.

108. Apelt S, Emrich HM. Sodium valproate in benzodiazepine withdrawal. Am J Psychiatry 1990;147(7):950–1.

109. Himmerich H, Nickel T, Dalal MA, et al. [Gabapentin treatment in a female patient with panic disorder and adverse effects under carbamazepine during benzodiazepine withdrawal]. Psychiatr Prax 2007;34(2):93–4 [in German].

110. Swift RM. Topiramate for the treatment of alcohol dependence: initiating abstinence. Lancet 2003;361(9370):1666–7.

111. Croissant B, Grosshans M, Diehl A, et al. Oxcarbazepine in rapid benzodiazepine detoxification. Am J Drug Alcohol Abuse 2008;34(5):534–40.

112. Ashton H. The treatment of benzodiazepine dependence. Addiction 1994; 89(11):1535–41.

113. Heberlein A, Bleich S, Kornhuber J, et al. [Benzodiazepine dependence: causalities and treatment options]. Fortschr Neurol Psychiatr 2009;77(1):7–15 [in German].

114. Kiefer F. [Treatment of benzodiazepine dependence: new insights into an old problem]. Fortschr Neurol Psychiatr 2009;77(1):1 [in German].

115. Balbani AP, Montovani JC. Methods for smoking cessation and treatment of nicotine dependence. Braz J Otorhinolaryngol 2005;71(6):820–7.

116. Mihaltan F, Ulmeanu R, Râşnoveanu R, et al. [New perspectives in the treatment of nicotine dependence]. Pneumologia 2006;55(1):36–9 [in Romanian].

117. Ray R, Schnoll RA, Lerman C. Nicotine dependence: biology, behavior, and treatment. Annu Rev Med 2009;60:247–60.

118. Stead LF, Perera R, Bullen C, et al. Nicotine replacement therapy for smoking cessation. Cochrane Database Syst Rev 2008;1:CD000146.

119. Goldman J, Shytle RD, Sanberg PR. Adding behavioral therapy to medication for smoking cessation. JAMA 1999;281(21):1984–5.

120. Keating GM, Siddiqui MA. Varenicline: a review of its use as an aid to smoking cessation therapy. CNS Drugs 2006;20(11):945–60.

121. Nides M, Oncken C, Gonzales D, et al. Smoking cessation with varenicline, a selective alpha4beta2 nicotinic receptor partial agonist: results from a 7-week, randomized, placebo- and bupropion-controlled trial with 1-year follow-up. Arch Intern Med 2006;166(15):1561–8.

122. Fossati R, Apolone G, Negri E, et al. A double-blind, placebo-controlled, randomized trial of bupropion for smoking cessation in primary care. Arch Intern Med 2007;167(16):1791–7.

123. Ebbert JO, Croghan IT, Sood A, et al. Varenicline and bupropion sustained-release combination therapy for smoking cessation. Nicotine Tob Res 2009; 11(3):234–9.

124. Maldonado J, Spiegel D. Hypnosis. In: Tashman A, Kay J, Lieberman J, editors. Psychiatry. New York: Wiley; 2008. p. 1982–2026.

125. Patten CA, Martin JE, Myers MG, et al. Effectiveness of cognitive-behavioral therapy for smokers with histories of alcohol dependence and depression. J Stud Alcohol 1998;59(3):327–35.

126. Stead LF, Lancaster T. Group behaviour therapy programmes for smoking cessation. Cochrane Database Syst Rev 2005;2:CD001007.

127. Carpenter MJ, Hughes JR, Solomon LJ, et al. Both smoking reduction with nicotine replacement therapy and motivational advice increase future cessation among smokers unmotivated to quit. J Consult Clin Psychol 2004;72(3):371–81.

128. Lai DT, Cahill K, Qin Y, et al. Motivational interviewing for smoking cessation. Cochrane Database Syst Rev 2010;1:CD006936.

An Approach to the Patient with Multiple Physical Symptoms or Chronic Disease

Janna S. Gordon-Elliott, MD[a,b], Philip R. Muskin, MD[b,c,d],*

KEYWORDS

- Chronic disease • Sick role • Denial • Somatoform disorders
- Conversion • Factitious • Hypochondriasis

Physicians practice under the assumption that patients see them because of physical or emotional distress, and for their expertise in diagnosing and treating their suffering. Patients follow physicians' recommendations to return to the pre-illness state. However, life is never this simple, which helps explain why the practice of medicine is an art. Doctors are comfortable with and define what a disease is (ie, a pathologic condition associated with pathophysiologic processes and observable lesions that affects a physical system). Disease is merely a component of the experience of illness. Illness is the response to a disease as perceived by individual patients (determined partly by their personality, social environment, experience, and world-view) and the people in their lives.[1]

This article discusses mismatches between illness and disease that emerge in the patient–physician relationship during the treatment of chronic diseases. Nowhere is the mismatch greater than in somatoform disorders, a group of conditions manifested by chronic symptoms without a clear connection to a "real" disease. This article examines challenges in the treatment of chronic conditions that are influenced by patients' behavior, circumstances, and sense of their illness.

The authors have nothing to disclose in relation to this manuscript.

[a] New York State Psychiatric Institute, New York-Presbyterian Hospital, Columbia University Medical Center, New York, NY, USA

[b] Division of Consultation-Liaison Psychiatry, Department of Psychiatry, New York-Presbyterian Hospital, Columbia University Medical Center, 622 West 168th Street, Mailbox #427, New York, NY 10032, USA

[c] Department of Psychiatry, Columbia University College of Physicians and Surgeons, New York, NY, USA

[d] Columbia University Psychoanalytic Center for Research and Training, New York, NY, USA

* Corresponding author. Division of Consultation-Liaison Psychiatry, Department of Psychiatry, New York-Presbyterian Hospital, Columbia University Medical Center, 622 West 168th Street, Mailbox #427, New York, NY 10032.

E-mail address: prm1@columbia.edu

Med Clin N Am 94 (2010) 1207–1216

doi:10.1016/j.mcna.2010.08.007

0025-7125/10/$ – see front matter © 2010 Elsevier Inc. All rights reserved.

medical.theclinics.com

MISMATCH #1: FAILURE TO ADOPT THE SICK ROLE

Mr A, a 48-year-old man, was recently diagnosed with type 2 diabetes mellitus. He made physician appointments because his wife convinced him to do so. He listened to the doctor when she talked about the importance of glucose control, nutrition, and exercise, but he did not seem to hear what she said. He left his glucose monitor in the closet and used it only once; his hemoglobin A1c was 9. Although he ate a balanced dinner, he often snacked on chips and soda.

In the vignette above, Mr A had difficulty adapting to the sick role. He did not want to view himself as "sick," or to assume the obligations of the sick role (eg, follow a prescribed diet and monitor his glucose).

Effective medical practice relies on an agreement between the doctor and the patient: the patient seeks help from the doctor for a condition; the condition has an underlying pathophysiologic mechanism that the physician seeks to understand and uses to direct appropriate treatment; and the patient complies with treatment and communicates any needs directly. The patient and doctor play their respective roles. For the patient, the sick role embodies two rights and two duties.[2] The "rights" include exemption from usual responsibilities and freedom from blame for being sick or being expected to recover without help. The "duties" or obligations dictate that the sick person should strive to get well and should accomplish this by seeking appropriate help and complying with recommendations of medical professionals. In this model the patient and doctor work collaboratively against the disease process, which is the obstacle. However, as medicine is a discipline that involves human beings, the parties inevitably stray from the script.

Among life stressors, "personal injury or illness" ranks sixth.[3] Patients are faced with several stressors associated with acute illness, including the physiologic effects of the disease and psychosocial issues (eg, fear of disability and death, impaired function in one's occupation and community, financial burdens, shifting responsibilities in one's family and community). When facing and surviving acute illness, patients must complete three successive stages: acknowledgment of illness, acceptance of dependency on others for necessary care, and return to normal function.[4]

As acuity of the illness subsides and a disease becomes chronic, adjustment to the sick role is fraught with challenges (eg, acceptance of indefinite illness and treatment without end). For a condition such as diabetes, this may mean countless painful finger pricks, changes in diet that may affect one's interactions with friends and family, numerous medication trials, and a fear that, regardless of how well it is managed, the disease may still result in morbidity and mortality. At various points along this process of accepting and confronting illness, patients struggle. They may choose to minimize what the doctor is telling them about their illness and the need for ongoing monitoring and treatment. They may become angry or depressed. Some seek help outside of the patient–doctor relationship (eg, through using the Internet for medical advice and treatment) and devalue their physician's care.[5]

The physician plays an integral role in the patient's acceptance of the sick role through allowing the patient to express concerns, by making room for mourning of the loss of a healthy life, and by helping the patient reclaim a sense of control. A patient's behavior, compliance with treatment, and self-care affects outcome. For Mr A, this would involve his taking charge of his diet, activity, and glucose control.

MISMATCH #2: FAILURE TO ADHERE TO RECOMMENDATIONS

On Dr X's initial visit with Mr B, a 39-year-old man, a blood pressure of 150/90 mm Hg was noted. Mr B acknowledged that it is "always high at the doctor's," and shrugged off the finding. Over the next couple of months, Mr B's blood pressure remained high and he resisted making any changes in diet or activity, Dr X recommended medication, but Mr B said, "It's not a big deal." As an afterthought, he added that he was on "some pill" a few years earlier, which caused erectile dysfunction, so he stopped the treatment.

Years of scientific research and huge sums of money go into the design and implementation of treatments for diseases. However, even the most advanced interventions are ineffective unless the patient takes them (as with Mr B). Untreated hypertension contributes significantly to inordinate health care expenditures and loss of productivity.[6] Because of hypertension's often-asymptomatic nature before end-organ damage has developed, many are unaware of their condition or are reluctant to follow a prescribed treatment.[7] Noncompliance with treatment across all medical conditions is somewhere in the range of 50%.[8] Factors such as access to care, coverage for visits and medications, and deficient public awareness of medical issues impact patients' ability to comply with proven medical treatments. However, a significant proportion of nonadherence to medical care is not a direct result of these system factors but rather a function of patients' choices not to comply.

The patient-related aspects of treatment noncompliance (eg, refusal to follow a doctor's recommendations) can strike physicians as particularly bewildering and distressing. Physicians assume that accurate diagnosis and access to treatment are the main obstacles to managing and curing disease; however, patients' choices to be nonadherent with treatment do not fit with this schema. Clearly, treatment can only work if a patient actually takes it. Therefore, after diagnosis and a review of management options, physicians must understand a patient's experience of treatment and the factors that impede treatment adherence.

With a condition such as hypertension (with few, if any, early symptoms), treatment side effects are often more bothersome to the patient than the illness. Unfortunately, in our vignette, Mr B reported experiencing sexual dysfunction in association with use of an antihypertensive medication, likely a β-blocker, but only after Dr X recommended treatment. Fatigue, dizziness, or erectile dysfunction may feel immediately distressing, whereas the possibility of long-term cardiovascular problems may feel much less salient. Treatment for other systemic illnesses, such as HIV infection, may impose lifestyle changes, such as taking a bevy of pills each day and coping with medication side effects (including lipodystrophy from protease inhibitors, and metabolic or cognitive changes).[9] Cancer treatments (eg, surgery, chemotherapy, radiation therapy) might continue for several years, with stretches of watchful-waiting. These treatments, although potentially life-saving, can have adverse effects, and the severity of these effects depend on the type of treatment and the meaning of the cancer and treatment to the patient. Chemotherapy might cause fatigue, nausea, and decline in libido, whereas a mastectomy and hair loss might result in feelings of being unattractive, undesirable, and unloved.

Depending on several factors inherent to the treatment and make-up of the patient, side effects can be highly variable and complex. It behooves doctors to explore the meaning of treatment to patients and their fears about, and responses to, treatment. In chronic illness, in which the goal is long-term management rather than cure, attention to these considerations (eg, "lifelong imprisonment" to treatment, concern about loss of autonomy) leads to more consistent management and a significantly better outcome.[9,10] Open communication throughout every stage of treatment facilitates the patient–physician alliance, which is as important in terms of overall outcome as is the selection of a therapeutic agent or intervention.

MISMATCH #3: FAILURE TO ACKNOWLEDGE ILLNESS: DENIAL

Ms C, a 56-year-old married woman with hypertension, noticed a lump in her breast, which she assumed was a product of her imagination. She did not have a primary care provider, because she always considered herself "healthy as a horse." She tried not to think about the lump and avoided touching her breast for more than a month. She did not tell her husband about the lump and pushed his hand away when he attempted to touch her breasts during intercourse.

Denial, a defense mechanism used to protect from overwhelming anxiety, serves to shut out frightening or otherwise potentially dangerous aspects of reality by disregarding the facts, such as that a disease exists or that treatment is needed. Denial comes to the attention of primary care physicians when a patient refuses to acknowledge a medical finding, to undergo further evaluation, or to accept clearly efficacious treatment.[11] In the above vignette, despite a worrisome finding, Ms C attempted to keep the idea that this might be cancer out of her own, and of others', awareness.

Denial is common when people are faced with a medical illness, and can have significant consequences. In one study of patients with ischemic heart disease being consented for treatment, 10% showed a significant impairment in their awareness of their condition and the acuity of the situation.[12] In another study of psychiatric consultations in a community hospital, 2.5% of all patients showed maladaptive denial of medical illness (defined as refusal of care because of a denial of illness or the seriousness of the illness).[11,13] Denial is different from a patient's stalwart optimism (in which, although aware of serious illness, there is perseverance with treatment) or refusal of treatment because of concerns about the risks of treatment or from underlying cognitive or psychiatric dysfunction.[14,15]

Beyond contributing to poor adherence with medical treatment, denial may challenge a doctor's notion of the practice of medicine and lead to confusion, anger, or helplessness. The patient's response to illness often seems unreasonable; in many cases, denial raises the question of the patient's capacity to make decisions related to treatment. Denial can also present more subtly (eg, manifest through missed appointments, intermittent medication nonadherence, or neglect of pursuing social services) and suggest the need for psychiatric consultation. Physicians can work effectively with patients who utilize denial.[16] The goal of the physician's intervention is to help the patient manage anxiety, while also reducing the risk of morbidity and mortality due to the medical illness; as long as the patient understands and appreciates the facts, the doctor can help the patient separate the belief in the diagnosis and need for treatment from the *fear* of the disease and treatment. A reasonable intervention might include saying: "I am not here to talk to you about having anything done. I would like to understand what is so frightening for you."[13] A nonthreatening and nonjudgmental stance can help the patient feel supported and safe, and allow for a dialogue about ongoing care. Careful assessment of the patient's awareness of the condition and the risks and benefits of the treatment (possibly aided by psychiatric consultation) can aid in the assessment and management of these complicated cases.

MISMATCH #4: PSYCHIATRIC COMORBIDITY

Mr D, a 36-year-old man with stable HIV infection diagnosed 7 years earlier, consistently used his medications and attended to provided self-care. Despite medication side effects, he maintained a good working relationship with his internist. Over the past 2 months, he started to skip medication doses. He failed to return phone calls from his physician regarding check-ups and blood tests. He isolated himself from friends, began having difficulty sleeping, and lost weight. At his next medical appointment he stated that he stopped his medications, impulsively used intravenous heroin for the first time in 8 years, and felt that he would rather die than continue with treatment.

In the above vignette, Mr D seemed to have depression and be neglected his health; he is not reluctant to accept being sick, as was the case with Mr B. Mr D may be choosing to give in to the disease because of the hopelessness associated with major depression.

While coping with chronic illness is challenging for emotionally healthy individuals, having a psychiatric illness adds another layer of complexity to the experience of illness and to the doctor–patient relationship. For example, psychiatric signs and symptoms are common in patients with chronic medical illness; having transient symptoms of anxiety and depression are understandable in reaction to a diagnosis, especially if it carries with it the potential for chronicity, morbidity, and mortality.[17] When symptoms persist and lead to marked distress that is out of proportion to what would be expected, or causes impairment in function, the patient may meet criteria for a diagnosis of adjustment disorder with depressed mood, with anxiety, or with mixed anxiety and depressed mood. Many chronic illnesses are associated with psychiatric symptoms and conditions (eg, depression, psychosis, mania, cognitive disorders, substance abuse, personality disorders, thoughts of suicide).[18–24]

Occasionally it is difficult to tease out the extent to which any psychiatric disorder was a risk factor for the development of that disease (through unhealthy habits or a lack of preventative care) or evolved as a consequence of the illness (through the direct effects of the disease, the psychological struggles with a serious chronic illness, or as a consequence of its biologic treatments). Having an Axis I diagnosis (eg, mood disorder, psychotic disorder, substance abuse disorder, cognitive disorder), an Axis II personality disorder, or maladaptive personality traits increases the likelihood that the patient will have an impaired alliance with a provider, difficulty complying appropriately with recommended treatment, and worse overall outcome than would a patient without a psychiatric disorder.[23,25,26] Psychiatric disorders influence how a patient views medical illness and pursues care, which can be challenging for the physician and may generate emotional reactions (eg, despair, anger).

To assess comorbid psychiatric illness, physicians can use validated measures (such as the Primary Care Evaluation of Mental Disorders [PRIME-MD] or the self-report version, the Patient Health Questionnaire [PHQ]).[27,28] A physician's uncharacteristically strong emotional reaction (either overly positive or negative) to a patient can be a clue that the patient may have a personality disorder.[29] A psychiatric consultation or the involvement of another trusted colleague may be indicated when the primary physician suspects that a psychiatric issue is adversely impacting a patient's medical care.

MISMATCH #5: OVERIDENTIFICATION WITH THE SICK ROLE

Ms E, a 43-year-old woman with a history of endometriosis, atopic dermatitis, fibromyalgia, and irritable bowel syndrome went to her primary care doctor monthly with concerns about her health. She described multiple physical complaints referable to different organs, and routinely requested tests and further evaluations, which were unrevealing. She often left out important information (such as her use of herbal remedies), and became angry easily when attempts were made to reassure her that she was healthy and that there was no cause for concern.

This final section discusses patients who perceive themselves as "sick" in the absence of adequate objective medical findings. These patients turn the sick role upside down in asserting that they are physically ill although the doctor has not found a disease to explain the symptoms.

Ms E violated the sick role by not being ill but nonetheless demanding that her physician experience her this way. With a somatoform disorder, the patient identifies symptoms suggestive of a general medical condition that cannot be fully explained by an underlying medical process. Ms E seems to suffer from somatization disorder. As defined by the text-revised fourth edition of the *Diagnostic and Statistical Manual of Mental Disorders* (*DSM-IV-TR*), patients with this disorder have multiple physical complaints that are not a direct result of a general medical condition, or, for patients who have a related general medical condition, their degree of impairment exceeds that which would be expected from the medical findings. The patient must, at some point during the course of the disorder, experience four pain symptoms, two gastrointestinal symptoms, one sexual symptom, and one neurologic symptom, other than pain. The patient does not intentionally feign the symptoms, and the onset must be before age 30 years. A less-severe form of the disorder in which patients have at least one physical complaint but not as many as in somatization disorder is known as *undifferentiated somatoform disorder*.[30]

In conversion disorder, symptoms or deficits of voluntary motor or sensory function that would seem to be caused by a neurologic or other general medical condition are reported, but they cannot be fully explained by a disease process after appropriate investigation. The patient neither consciously nor intentionally produces the symptoms. Underlying psychological processes precipitate or exacerbate the symptoms. Nevertheless, the reaction of physicians to these patients often includes disbelief that the symptoms are not intentionally produced; anger is often directed toward the patient. Symptoms of conversion disorder cannot be limited to pain or sexual dysfunction, and the presentation of a conversion disorder cannot be explained by a culturally sanctioned behavior or experience (eg, as in amok, or falling-out/blackout).[30]

Hypochondriasis is manifest through preoccupation with having a serious disease based on misinterpretations of otherwise normal bodily sensations or signals. Afflicted patients are not reassured by appropriate medical evaluations that disprove the presence of the disease. Unlike somatization disorder (in which the patient has the experience of being ill), the hypochondriacal patient fears being ill. In hypochondriasis, the concern about medical illness is not of delusional intensity; that is, the person is able to entertain the possibility that it is "all in my head" but remains preoccupied with the concern. If the concerns become delusional, the symptom would be more appropriately classified as a delusional disorder, somatic type, or as part of another psychotic condition. The fear of being ill cannot be better explained by an anxiety disorder, a mood disorder, or another somatoform disorder. The worry about having a disease causes significant distress or impairment, and lasts at least 6 months. Patients with hypochondriasis can, over a lifetime, develop numerous different hypochondriacal preoccupations, often with a waxing and waning course.[30]

Somatoform disorder not otherwise specified (NOS) is a diagnostic category that includes disorders with physical symptoms (eg, pseudocyesis, in which the patient has a false belief of being pregnant) that do not fulfill criteria for any specific somatoform disorder, or a disorder characterized by somatic or hypochondriacal symptoms that does not otherwise fit under another diagnostic classification, because of either reduced severity or the duration of symptoms.[30]

Factitious disorder involves an individual's overidentification with and attempt to occupy the sick role. In factitious disorder (the most severe form of which is known as *Munchausen syndrome*), the patient intentionally produces symptoms (in contrast to conversion disorder, in which the symptoms are unconsciously driven) with the goal of assuming the sick role and obtaining the privileges that it confers. This condition is distinguished from malingering, in which the patient consciously feigns a condition for a secondary gain (eg, time off work, financial reward, avoidance of legal troubles). Factitious disorder can involve the production of either physical or psychological symptoms, but the goal remains the same: to become a patient.[30]

Physicians often find it frustrating when a patient does not assume the sick role easily, but more troubling for physicians is when a patient seeks out the sick role because of underlying an psychological need. In somatoform disorders and factitious disorder, the psychological need for the sick role is the cause of the disorder. Doctors may view these patients as enraging, curious, or even pathetic.

Patients with other psychiatric disorders may also display similar patterns of overidentification with the sick role while more subtly still eliciting physician disquiet. Roughly 30% to 60% of patients in primary care settings present with physical complaints with no identifiable organic basis.[31] Patients with generalized anxiety disorder, defined by having at least 6 months of excessive anxiety and worry along with several physical symptoms, may be excessively concerned about illness or death. In panic disorder, patients experience acute episodes characterized by intense physical symptoms that are interpreted as serious, even life-threatening, medical conditions. Major depressive disorder often presents with significant anxiety and somatic preoccupations, sometimes reaching delusional proportions. Patients with psychotic disorders (eg, schizophrenia, delusional disorder) may have delusional beliefs about having a serious medical illness. Patients with underlying psychiatric disorders and multiple unexplained physical symptoms may not be reassured despite exhaustive evaluations and testing. Patients with borderline personality disorder, who have difficulty regulating their mood and maintaining interpersonal stability, may complain of multiple physical complaints as a proxy for psychological distress, and become angry when their doctors, after reasonable medical investigation, find no evidence of physical disease. Patients with a dependent personality disorder, to satisfy needs for attachment and prevent potential abandonment, often cite multiple physical problems with the goal of keeping the physician interested and involved.[25]

Individuals without an active psychiatric condition can also rely on the sick role for emotional sustenance, especially during periods of stress or acute crisis; for example, the patients with HIV-infection who has minimal social support may become reliant on her medical providers and invested in her identity as a patient, or the patient with Hodgkin lymphoma may, after full remission, struggle to readjust to the role of a healthy person and delay returning to work, or tell his spouse that he is "just not ready" to start a family. Such patients may seek frequent appointments or proffer requests that seem unnecessary or even demanding (eg, obtaining expensive medical testing or extended medical disability). Physicians may become overwhelmed by a patient's neediness, or become resentful that one patient is taking up so much time that could be spent on "sicker" patients. Moreover, physicians may get frustrated that a patient is using medical care to treat emotional needs.

How can busy physicians with many competing demands respond to these patients? Perhaps most important is to modify their conceptualization of the patient. These patients depend psychologically, to varying degrees, on the identity of being sick. For them, it is often more acceptable or effective to exhibit emotional distress than physical symptoms. The extent to which these patients are aware that they are behaving in this manner, or even that they are suffering psychologically, varies. These patients rely on medical caretakers for their emotional requirements. By being available and responsive, the physician serves a vital role. Sometimes that awareness is itself enough to lessen the sense of burden and frustration that these patients can engender in their health care providers.

Practical pointers for physicians who care for patients with somatoform disorders include setting fair limits around the frequency of visits and other forms of communication, consistently reinforcing clinical indications for tests and procedures, and focusing the patient during visits. Asking (at the beginning of the appointment) which symptom the patient wants to discuss during the visit, while acknowledging that this may be only one of many concerns, can be containing and reassuring. When appropriate, the physician can encourage the patient to talk about the concerns or beliefs that might contribute to a reluctance to give up medical symptoms. For example, "I worry I won't perform as well at work as I did before," or "I am not a capable mother; if I improve and my husband returns to work, I won't be able to cope."

Making efforts to empathize with the patient's experience and to learn about who this person *is* (as opposed to what the patient *has*) can help the physician who feels frustrated or helpless with a patient. Although reassurance and support are useful, a patient will not benefit from hearing "the symptoms are all in your head."[32] Just as it is important not to miss the psychological component of physical symptoms, it is imperative that evidence of psychological dysfunction does not blind the physician to the presence of an underlying physical illness. In one series of psychiatric outpatients, 9% had medical illnesses producing psychiatric symptoms.[33]

When a psychiatric illness is suspected, the physician should consider obtaining a psychiatric consultation. Using the PRIME-MD or PHQ may help in evaluating a psychiatric disorder.[27,28] For a patient who is invested in being viewed as medically ill, it is essential for the medical provider, when recommending a psychiatric evaluation, to frame it as an adjunct to the current treatment. The physician should reinforce that the primary care relationship will not end when the patient sees a psychiatrist. These patients are particularly sensitive to feelings of abandonment; without special attention to this dynamic, the patient may experience the request for consultation as rejection and choose instead to terminate all care.[32]

Patients with factitious illness or conversion disorder, perhaps because of their particular difficulty in tolerating distress, require a more specialized approach. To make either diagnosis, all relevant medical conditions must first be ruled out. For patients thought to have factitious disorder, strict limits must be placed on invasive testing in the absence of objective physical findings. When conversion disorder is suspected, confirmation of the diagnosis may be facilitated by use of hypnosis or benzodiazepines to reduce the patient's inhibitions and to resolve symptoms. These individuals benefit from reassurance and frequent monitoring during the acute presentation of symptoms, with suggestive comments such as "these sorts of things generally resolve in a few hours." For patients with either conversion disorder or factitious illness, confrontation about the production of symptoms rarely works. Psychiatric consultation is almost always indicated when either of these disorders is suspected. Supportive measures, such as scheduling regular visits, encourage the patient to see that the therapeutic relationship does not need to rely on the production (conscious or unconscious) of symptoms. In both conditions it is useful to connect the emotional needs of the patient with the production of a physical symptom, emphasizing how somatization is an understandable but maladaptive way of dealing with life.[34,35]

SUMMARY

The patient and physician, although ideally working together against disease, may not always see eye-to-eye in their understanding of, and approach to, sickness, suffering, and recovery. In the management of chronic medical conditions, physicians and patients may disagree on the meaning of illness and the experience of treatment. Illness presents a patient with a crisis; it may also be an opportunity for tremendous growth and change.[9] The physician can play a meaningful role for a patient faced with sickness. Looking beyond the disease and into the patient's experience of illness can be a vital step toward joining the patient and moving cooperatively toward enhanced health and well-being. In somatoform disorders and related conditions, the patient presents with an illness experience, but the physician understands that the patient has a psychiatric disorder. Physicians frequently have strong negative reactions to patients when these mismatches arise; unfortunately, these reactions adversely influence treatment. By being aware of common pitfalls and challenging dynamics, physicians may adapt and respond in a more helpful manner.

REFERENCES

1. Eisenberg L. Disease and illness: distinctions between professional and popular ideas of sickness. Cult Med Psychiatry 1977;1:9–23.
2. Parsons T. The social system. New York: Free Press; 1951.
3. Holmes TH, Rahe RH. The social readjustment rating scale. J Psychosom Res 1967;11:213–8.
4. Perry S, Viederman M. Management of emotional reactions to acute medical illness. Med Clin North Am 1981;65:3–14.
5. Diaz JA, Griffith RA, Ng JJ, et al. Patients' use of the internet for medical information. J Gen Intern Med 2002;17:180–5.
6. Lawes CM, Vander Hoorn S, Law MR, et al. Blood pressure and the global burden of disease 2000. Part II: estimates of attributable burden. J Hypertens 2006;24: 423–30.
7. Hajjar I, Kotchen TA. Trends in prevalence, awareness, treatment, and control of hypertension in the United States, 1988–2000. JAMA 2003;290:199–206.
8. Dunbar-Jacob J, Mortimer-Stephens MK. Treatment adherence in chronic disease. J Clin Epidemiol 2001;54:S57–60.
9. Nields JA, Grimaldi JA. Infectious diseases. In: Schein LA, Bernard HS, Spitz HI, et al, editors. Psychosocial treatment for medical conditions. New York: Brunner-Routledge; 2003. p. 267–332.
10. Gazzola LR, Muskin PR. The impact of stress and the objectives of psychosocial interventions. In: Schein LA, Bernard HS, Spitz HI, et al, editors. Psychosocial treatment for medical conditions. New York: Brunner-Routledge; 2003. p. 373–406.
11. Strauss DH, Spitzer RL, Muskin PR. Maladaptive denial of physical illness: a proposal for DSM-IV. Am J Psychiatry 1990;147:1168–72.
12. Appelbaum PS, Grisso T. Capacities of hospitalized, medically ill patients to consent to treatment. Psychosomatics 1997;38:119–25.
13. Muskin PR, Feldhammer T, Gelfand JL, et al. Maladaptive denial of physical illness: a useful new "diagnosis". Int J Psychiatry Med 1998;28:463–77.
14. Druss GR, Douglas CJ. Adaptive response to illness and disability. Gen Hosp Psychiatry 1988;10:163–8.
15. Shelp EE, Perl M. Denial in clinical medicine: a reexamination of the concept and its significance. Arch Intern Med 1985;145:697–9.
16. Kornfeld DS, Muskin PR, Tahil FA. A review of requests for psychiatric evaluation of mental capacity in the general hospital: a significant teaching opportunity. Psychosomatics 2009;50:468–73.

17. Derogatis LR, Feldstein M, Morrow G, et al. A survey of psychotropic drug prescriptions in an oncology population. Cancer 1979;44:1919–29.
18. Angelino AF, Treisman GJ. Issues in co-morbid severe mental illnesses in HIV infected individuals. Int Rev Psychiatry 2008;20:95–101.
19. Breitbart WS, Alici Y. Psycho-oncology. Harv Rev Psychiatry 2009;17:361–76.
20. Frankenburg FR, Zanarini MC. Personality disorders and medical comorbidity. Curr Opin Psychiatry 2006;19:428–31.
21. Goodwin R, Marusic A, Hoven C. Suicide attempts in the United States: the role of physical illness. Soc Sci Med 2003;56:1783–8.
22. Iacovides A, Siamouli M. Comorbid mental and somatic disorders: an epidemiological perspective. Curr Opin Psychiatry 2008;21:417–21.
23. Prince M, Patel V, Saxena S, et al. No health without mental health. Lancet 2007; 370:859–77.
24. Shapiro PA. Psychiatric aspects of cardiovascular disease. Psychiatr Clin North Am 1996;19:613–29.
25. Groves MS, Muskin PR. Psychological responses to illness. In: Levinson JL, editor. Textbook of psychosomatic medicine. Washington, DC: American Psychiatric Publishing; 2005. p. 67–88.
26. Ingersoll KS, Cohen J. The impact of medication regimen factors on adherence to chronic treatment: a review of literature. J Behav Med 2008;31:213–24.
27. Spitzer RL, Kroenke K, Linzer M, et al. Health-related quality of life in primary care patients with mental disorders. Results from the PRIME-MD 1000 Study. JAMA 1995;274:1511–7.
28. Spitzer RL, Kroenke K, Williams JB. Validation and utility of a self-report version of PRIME-MD: the PHQ primary care study. Primary care evaluation of mental disorders. Patient health questionnaire. JAMA 1999;282:1737–44.
29. Haas LJ, Leiser JP, Magill MK, et al. Management of the difficult patient. Am Fam Physician 2005;72:2063–8.
30. American Psychiatric Association. Diagnostic and statistical manual of mental disorders. Text Revision. 4th edition. Washington, DC: American Psychiatric Association; 2000. p. 485–517.
31. Kirmayer L, Robbins J. Three forms of somatization in primary care: prevalence, co-occurrence, and sociodemographic characteristics. J Nerv Ment Dis 179: 647–655.
32. Muskin PR, Mirasol EG. Physical signs and symptoms. In: Tasman A, Kay J, TLieberman J, editors. Psychiatry. 3rd edition. Hoboken (NJ): John Wiley & Sons, Ltd; 2008. p. 621–33.
33. Hall RC, Popkin MK, Devaul R, et al. Physical illness presenting as psychiatric disease. Arch Gen Psychiatry 1978;35:1315–20.
34. Abbey SE. Somatization and somatoform disorders. In: Levinson JL, editor. Textbook of psychosomatic medicine. Washington, DC: American Psychiatric Publishing; 2005. p. 271–96.
35. Ford CV. Deception syndromes: factitious disorders and malingering. In: Levinson JL, editor. Textbook of psychosomatic medicine. Washington, DC: American Psychiatric Publishing; 2005. p. 297–309.

An Approach to Symptoms at the Interface of Medicine and Psychiatry: Pain, Insomnia, Weight Loss and Anorexia, Fatigue and Forgetfulness, and Sexual Dysfunction

Oliver Freudenreich, MD, FAPM[a,b,c,*], Nicholas Kontos, MD[d,e], Shamim H. Nejad, MD[a,d,c], Anne F. Gross, MD[a,d]

KEYWORDS

• Symptoms • Pain • Insomnia • Weight loss • Fatigue
• Sexual dysfunction

Primary care physicians commonly see patients who have somatic complaints for which no clear organic etiology can be found. For example, Bridges and Goldberg[1] estimated that 20% of new primary care visits were for unexplained physical symptoms. In an analysis of almost 14,000 community dwellers, Kroenke and Price[2] found that somatic symptoms were not only prevalent and problematic but unexplained in one-third of cases and were associated with an increased likelihood of psychiatric disorders.

Oliver Freudenreich, MD, has received research grant support from Pfizer. The other authors have nothing to disclose.
[a] Harvard Medical School, 25 Shattuck Street, Boston, MA 02115, USA
[b] Infectious Disease Psychiatric Consultation Service, Division of Psychiatry and Medicine, Department of Medicine, Massachusetts General Hospital, 55 Fruit Street, Boston, MA 02114, USA
[c] Division of Psychiatry and Medicine, Department of Psychiatry, Massachusetts General Hospital, 55 Fruit Street, Boston, MA 02114, USA
[d] Department of Psychiatry, Massachusetts General Hospital, 55 Fruit Street, Boston, MA 02114, USA
[e] Department of Psychiatry, Harvard Medical School, Boston, MA, USA
* Corresponding author. Freedom Trail Clinic, 25 Staniford Street, Boston, MA 02114.
E-mail address: ofreudenreich@partners.org

Med Clin N Am 94 (2010) 1217–1227
doi:10.1016/j.mcna.2010.08.006
0025-7125/10/$ – see front matter © 2010 Elsevier Inc. All rights reserved.

The article discusses how a psychiatrist thinks about a patient who presents with a specific somatic complaint for which a medical work-up has failed to uncover an etiology, and focusses on several somatic symptoms that each can be a prominent symptom of depression (eg, pain, insomnia, weight loss and loss of appetite, fatigue and forgetfulness, or sexual dysfunction), which is perhaps the most important psychiatric diagnosis to make in this context. It concludes with the management of patients for whom no satisfactory medical or psychiatric diagnosis can be made.

PSYCHIATRIC APPROACH TO SOMATIC SYMPTOMS

When a patient seeks consultation, the chief complaint needs to be understood (with regards to its exact nature, its onset and time course, and its aggravating and relieving factors). The presenting complaint, however, might not be the most useful symptom to determine the diagnosis. Obtaining a full review of systems is often quite important. This review of systems should cover not only the present problems but include a lifetime review of somatic symptoms and medical diagnoses, particularly for which no medical explanation was found. Well-validated instruments (like the Patient Health Questionnaire [PHQ]-15) can help identify symptoms not initially reported.[3] The goal of such a comprehensive review is to identify psychiatric syndromes or diagnoses for which specific treatment (eg, psychopharmacological, psychological, or cognitive–behavioral) can make a substantial difference. Of these conditions, the most common are a somatized presentation secondary to major depression or anxiety disorders (eg, panic disorder).[4] An important, albeit rare, consideration is psychosis that presents with somatic complaints.

Depression and Somatic Symptoms

Depression is a disorder that encompasses more than mere sadness. In addition to its psychological symptoms, physical signs are an integral part of the illness.[5] Aches and pains, a lack of energy, disrupted sleep, a change in appetite, and palpitations are common bodily complaints in depressed individuals.[6] The number of somatic symptoms experienced predicts the presence of depression.[7] The terms masked depression or depression sine depression capture the essence of a depressed patient who presents with predominantly somatic complaints. In a World Health Organization study (conducted in 14 countries on 5 continents), half of the depressed patients had multiple unexplained medical symptoms, and 11% of them denied psychological symptoms of depression.[8]

Depression is not a default diagnosis for a patient with unexplained medical symptoms when nothing else can be found. With careful questioning, a criteria-based diagnosis of major depressive disorder (MDD) is often established. An approach that normalizes the content and style of the distressed patient may overcome obstacles when considering a diagnosis of depression.[6] In the event that a treatment trial is undertaken in the absence of a confirmed psychiatric diagnosis, a clearly defined end point is crucial, as is a plan to stop the intervention if it is ineffective.

PSYCHIATRIC APPROACH TO SPECIFIC SOMATIC SYMPTOMS
Pain

Epidemiology and assessment
The International Association for the Study of Pain (IASP) defines pain as "an unpleasant sensory and emotional experience associated with actual or potential tissue damage or described in terms of such damage."[9] This definition recognizes that pain has both an acute nociceptive aspect and an emotional–psychiatric dimension. Epidemiologic

studies indicate that the lifetime prevalence of pain symptoms is high, ranging from 24% to 37%.[10] In one European telephone survey, moderate-to-severe chronic pain affected 19% of adults queried.[11] Not surprisingly, chronic pain significantly impacts a patient's psychological well-being.[12]

All patients should be assessed for pain complaints as a matter of routine. Although pain is always a subjective experience, objective measurements of pain are possible; measures should include the severity of pain and its functional relevance.[13] Pain severity can be measured and monitored by means of a numerical rating scale or a visual analog scale. In addition, the physician should obtain a detailed history of when and how the pain began, of treatments received, and of the patient's relationships with current and past physicians. Furthermore, the patient's past and present mental state (including an assessment of suicidal thoughts) and the family's psychiatric history need to be explored. The question, "Do you feel like you are being punished?" may guide a clinician toward a diagnosis of a comorbid depression.

Differential diagnosis

Chronic pain and psychiatric disorders (particularly depression,[14] anxiety, and somatization disorder) are commonly comorbid. Bair and colleagues[15] reported that roughly two-thirds of patients with depression have one or more pain complaints and that depression occurs in up to 85% of patients with pain disorders. Anxiety disorders (usually generalized anxiety or panic disorder) are found in approximately one-third of patients with intractable pain. Somatoform disorders involve chronic complaints of, and anxiety about, physical illness. These complaints exist in the absence of objective organic findings to explain the pain. Visceral pain (eg, pain from the esophagus, abdomen, and pelvis) that is associated with psychiatric conditions, especially somatoform disorders, can create a diagnostic challenge.

Treatment

Several neurotransmitters (eg, serotonin, norepinephrine, dopamine) modulate pain via their actions in the periphery and in the central nervous system (CNS). The relief from pain obtained by use of antidepressants is often independent of their effects on mood and of their alleviation of MDD.[16,17] In particular, serotonin–noradrenergic reuptake inhibitors (SNRIs) seem to have particular efficacy in the treatment of chronic pain. Desipramine, a tricyclic antidepressant (TCA), has been shown to relieve pain in diabetic neuropathy (in both nondepressed and depressed patients),[18] and to relieve post-herpetic neuralgia.[19] Duloxetine, a SNRI, has become the first antidepressant to have a specific US Food and Drug Administration (FDA)-approved indication for the treatment of painful diabetic neuropathy.[20] Duloxetine also has been efficacious for pain reduction in fibromyalgia and for the reduction of tender points, stiffness scores, and increasing the tender point pain threshold when compared with placebo.[21] Nonpharmacologic approaches to pain treatment also may be incorporated into the treatment plan, particularly when medications are not fully effective, they result in unwanted side effects, or they fail to improve physical and emotional function. Studies have demonstrated that multidisciplinary, multimodal rehabilitation can reduce pain, improve function, and build self-efficacy.[22] In a meta-analysis of 25 psychosocial treatment interventions, Devine[23] demonstrated the utility of psychoeducational treatment, particularly, cognitive–behavioral therapy (CBT) that emphasized relaxation, support groups, and education for patients with cancer-related pain. The efficacy of CBT in the treatment of various pain complaints has been demonstrated in numerous studies and been reviewed in multiple meta-analyses.[24]

Insomnia

Epidemiology and assessment

Narrowly defined, insomnia (difficulty falling asleep or staying asleep, or having non-restorative sleep associated with daytime dysfunction or distress) lasting for more than 4 weeks affects 10% of adults in the United States.[25] Insomnia can be a primary condition or result from medical or psychiatric illnesses. Once the medical causes of insomnia have been ruled out, the evaluation should focus on the diagnosis of primary sleep disorders and on psychiatric and behavioral causes (eg, depression, anxiety, stress, drug use, poor sleep habits, and behavioral conditioning). The interview can be supplemented by standardized questionnaires (eg, via the Epworth Sleepiness Scale, [ESS]) to quantify the degree of daytime sleepiness, and by a 1-week sleep diary (to further characterize the nature of the sleep problem). A sleep diary can be helpful to uncover a circadian rhythm disorder in a patient who lacks a structured schedule and who complains about initial insomnia. Polysomnography (PSG) can facilitate diagnosis of obstructive sleep apnea (OSA) or periodic limb movements of sleep (PLMS). Because obese patients on maintenance psychotropics are at high risk for OSA (because these agents predispose to weight gain), a PSG should be considered.[26]

Differential diagnosis

Although most patients with insomnia do not have a psychiatric diagnosis, 40% do.[27] Depression accounts for most cases.[28] Sleep disturbances are not only a core feature of MDD,[29] but they are also a risk factor for the development of the first episode of depression.[30] New and intractable insomnia may be a harbinger of MDD. In addition, 70% of patients with successfully treated and remitted depression continue to experience sleep disturbances; this increases their risk for depression relapse.[31] Increasingly, the recognition and treatment of insomnia in partially remitted patients with depression are seen as important clinical goals.[32]

Treatment

The initial treatment of insomnia often focuses on the elimination of unproductive maneuvers (eg, spending excessive time in bed, taking long naps, or resorting to alcohol to facilitate sleep). The basic principles of sleep hygiene should be reviewed with the patient to guide interventions. For a motivated patient, CBT can effectively target maladaptive approaches to sleep and excessive anxiety about sleep.[33,34]

Unfortunately, the previously mentioned maneuvers are often ineffective, and agents used to promote sleep may disrupt it (eg, SNRIs have the potential to disrupt sleep microarchitecture).[35] Therefore, affected individuals with psychiatric comorbidities require targeted pharmacologic interventions. Sedating antidepressants (eg, trazodone[36]) frequently are administered in the absence of compelling data[37]; however, clinical trials have shown that the addition of a nonbenzodiazepine hypnotic (eg, zolpidem[38] or eszopiclone[39]) is effective in SSRI-treated patients with insomnia. Appropriate oversight of hypnotic prescriptions is a critical element of the care of psychiatric patients at risk for suicide. Using low-dose sedating second-generation antipsychotics (eg, quetiapine) for insomnia lacks support from clinical trials and carries the risk of metabolic complications.

In the subgroup of patients with depression and residual fatigue despite good sleep, stimulants (like modafinil) can be used successfully.[40,41] The management of treatment-resistant depression with methylphenidate or dexamphetamine usually requires care by a specialist.[42]

Weight Loss and Anorexia

Assessment

Once medical causes of weight loss have been examined and eliminated, attention should turn to psychiatric illnesses (with eating disorders [eg, anorexia nervosa], psychosis, and depression being key considerations). It is often helpful to ask if the weight loss is voluntary or involuntary. Voluntary weight loss occurs in patients who starve themselves (or who increase their exercise) to lose weight for health reasons but also in those who attempt to lose weight because of a distorted body image (eg, anorexia nervosa). A psychotic motivation related to avoiding food (eg, a fear of being poisoned) is another cause of voluntary weight loss. In a patient with either anorexia nervosa or psychosis, the reasons for starvation may not be immediately forthcoming, and the weight loss may appear involuntary. A complete weight history (with a food diary; calorie counts; and details of purging, exercise, and medication use [eg, diuretics, laxatives, ipecac syrup, and diet pills]) can help establish nonmedical causes of weight loss. In patients with anorexia nervosa, indifference to cachexia appears in stark contrast to appropriate concerns held by the medically ill.

Weight loss due to a loss of appetite is one of the hallmarks of melancholic depression. Particularly in an elderly individual, unexplained weight loss can be the main symptom of depression. In those with dementia, the loss of smell may be associated with the loss of appetite, and with subsequent weight loss. If weight loss occurs despite a sound appetite and sufficient sleep, depression is unlikely. In some elderly, the anorexia of aging with weight loss may result from simply not taking in enough calories.[43]

Few drugs cause sustained weight loss; however, dieting drugs and prescribed or illicit stimulants can account for weight loss. The antiepileptic drug, topiramate, frequently used for the prophylaxis of migraine headaches, reliably causes weight loss.[44]

Treatment

If weight loss is caused by depression, any antidepressant should normalize appetite and lead to weight gain. Mirtazapine, an antidepressant with effects on the histamine$_1$ and serotonin$_{2c}$ receptors, is a potent stimulator of appetite and weight gain[45]; it may even be effective in cancer-related weight loss.[46] Ongoing weight gain, however, can be problematic in the maintenance phase of depression treatment. Among the second-generation antidepressants, mirtazapine and paroxetine are most often linked with weight gain.[47] Low doses of stimulants can be used to enhance appetite and activate a withdrawn patient. This approach, in conjunction with nutritional support, can effectively treat cachexia–anorexia in an elderly patient.

Fatigue and Forgetfulness

Epidemiology and assessment

Fatigue is a significant complaint in up to 25% of the population.[2] It is frequently linked with cognitive inefficiency, and the International Classification of Disease (ICD)–10 recognizes this within its version of "neurasthenia" (which entails disproportionate fatigue with mental or physical effort).[48] Contrary to the ICD-10's exclusion criteria for this entity, psychopathology is apparent in about 45% of cases.[49] The importance of depression as a consideration in the assessment of fatigue and cognitive complaints is reflected in the popular, but ill-defined, concept of depressive pseudodementia.

Suspicion of depression should not wait for a fatigued patient's endorsements of dysphoria or stress, since they may be averse to psychiatric formulations.[50] Instead, for example, the activity-to-fatigue ratio may give hints as to a patient's level of motivation; withdrawal into sedentary hobbies, or exaggerated feelings of guilt over lapsed responsibilities can provide clinicians with evidence for a possible depressive syndrome. Memory complaints can be a catch-all phrase for cognitive disturbances. Screening with the Mini-Mental State Examination (MMSE) should be appended with categorical and multiple-choice prompts for the recall items. Correct cued answers suggest retrieval problems rather than the encoding deficit typical of Alzheimer dementia. Intact spontaneous recall of recent events hints at a motivational problem when performance on formal anterograde memory screens is poor.

Differential diagnosis

Many neuropsychiatric conditions are accompanied by fatigue and cognitive complaints. In addition to depression, anxiety disorders and stress are important considerations. Sleep deprivation due to a medical condition that interrupts sleep (eg, pain or frequent awakenings to urinate) or an overscheduled life can lead to fatigue. Sleep deprivation can be assessed by the propensity to fall asleep easily when given the opportunity (eg, sitting in the car). Dementia and delirium are covered elsewhere in this monograph. Substance abuse demands vigilance as do prescribed agents that can contribute to iatrogenically induced fatigue and cognitive dulling.

Treatment of fatigue

Fatigue and cognitive complaints are best treated by avoiding pharmaceuticals with CNS activity, particularly anticholinergic agents, pain medications, and benzodiazepines. Their use in any patient with ongoing fatigue or cognitive complaints should be minimized, albeit not at the cost of undertreatment of symptomatic psychiatric syndromes. Bupropion is frequently advocated as a stimulating antidepressant, although evidence for this is lacking. Use of modafinil and traditional psychostimulants was mentioned in the insomnia section. However, despite conclusive evidence of mental status disruption and fall risk, benzodiazepines[51] and anticholinergic agents continue to be administered to those with cognitive complaints.[52]

Sexual Dysfunction

Epidemiology and assessment

Approximately 40% of women and 30% of men in the United States experience sexual problems.[53] Women are most likely to report low sexual desire, while men are more likely to complain of premature ejaculation. Psychiatric illness (especially depression), and use of psychotropics (particularly serotonin reuptake inhibitors [SRIs]), are important contributors to sexual dysfunction.[54]

Most patients (and many physicians) are uncomfortable discussing sexual matters. "Are you presently satisfied with your sex life?" is a good screening question that, if asked nonjudgmentally as part of the medical history, can lead to further detailed inquiry about Kaplan's three phases of desire, excitement (arousal), and orgasm. Normalizing questions (eg, "Many patients taking antidepressants experience side effects; what about you?") invite patients to discuss concerns about medications (including medication-induced sexual dysfunction, which is a common reason for patients to discontinue treatment) that they might not have volunteered.[55] Psychological causes of sexual dysfunction include predisposing factors (eg, lack of experience or sexual trauma), precipitation factors (eg, problem in a partner), and maintaining factors (eg, stress, depression, or gender identity issues). Although many sexual disorders are related to psychological factors alone, organic factors must be excluded as they might either be directly responsible for the sexual dysfunction or cause secondary psychological reactions.

Erectile dysfunction and loss of desire

Patients with depression are more likely to suffer from sexual dysfunction than are those in the general population, with 40% to 50% of patients suffering from decreased sexual desire at baseline, before the initiation of an antidepressant.[56] In the Massachusetts Male Aging Study, patients with depression were 1.8 times more likely to have erectile dysfunction (ED) than those who were not depressed.[57] The relationship between sexual dysfunction appears to be related to the length and severity of the depressive episode. ED can have a negative impact on quality of life, can lead to poor coping and disease management, and may even lead to depression. Conversely, sildenafil treatment of ED has improved depression and quality of life.[58]

Many psychotropics (including antidepressants) can cause sexual dysfunction.[55] SRI-induced sexual dysfunction includes decreased libido and arousal, and delayed or absent ejaculation and orgasm; these are thought to be primarily related to agonism at the $5-HT_2$ receptor. Mirtazapine, which antagonizes $5-HT_2$, may be associated with a lower incidence and severity of sexual dysfunction as compared with SRIs.[59] Primary dopamine agonists (including psychostimulants and bupropion) are associated with much lower rates of sexual dysfunction. TCAs and monoamine oxidase inhibitors (MAOIs), both increase serotonin availability, and are therefore associated with high rates of sexual dysfunction.

Treatment of sexual dysfunction related to depression and its treatment

Commonly used strategies to treat SRI-induced sexual dysfunction include dose reduction, drug holidays, and antidote therapy using dopamine agonists (eg, psychostimulants, ropinirole, pramipexole, or bupropion) or the $alpha_2$-adrenergic receptor antagonist, yohimbine.[60] The phosphodiesterase-5-inhibitor, sildenafil, has been efficacious for the treatment of ED caused by depression or use of antidepressants in men[61,62] as well as for the treatment of SRI-associated sexual dysfunction in women.[63] A switch to bupropion as the antidepressant with the lowest risk for sexual side effects can also be effective.[55]

THE APPROACH TO NONREPSONSE TO PSYCHIATRIC TREATMENT

Earlier, there was discussion of an approach to patients whose somatic symptom is thought to be due to depression as one important and treatable psychiatric condition. When treatment of apparent depression does not ameliorate or resolve the somatic complaint, the internist should consider three other possibilities.

Partial Remission or Ineffective Treatment

Initial treatments often improve depressive symptoms without leading to a full remission; less often, but still frequent, they are ineffective. To optimize the treatment response, the internist should titrate prescriptions of first-line antidepressants, and initiate a second trial in a timely manner if the first agent is either intolerable or ineffective. In the Sequenced Trial to Relieve Depression (STAR*D) trial, two sequential trials achieved remission in about 50% of cases.[64]

Incorrect Diagnosis

If one assumes that a patient has been adherent with treatment, then lack of treatment response should trigger a diagnostic reassessment; this is especially true for conditions diagnosed on the basis of subjective complaints. Common depression look-alikes in psychiatry include substance use disorders, generalized anxiety disorder, post-traumatic stress disorder, bipolar depression, and early dementia. Persistence of, or any change in, the index symptom also may mandate revisiting the somatic work-up. Clinicians should be wary of allowing depression (or any other psychiatric diagnosis) to too easily satisfy Occam's razor.[65]

Medically Unexplained Symptoms

Many somatic complaints defy medical explanation.[2] While the persistently suffering and impaired subset of patients with these symptoms often has comorbid psychopathology,[66] treating the underlying depression is ineffective unless clinical depression is present. For patients with an intense fear or preoccupation with their physical state, frequent brief scheduled visits with targeted physical examinations and avoidance of extraneous therapeutics and diagnostic testing comprise the standard of care.[67] This last element is critical for a patient committed to a fringe idea or for a person who is overidentified with a functional somatic syndrome (such as in fibromyalgia or chronic fatigue syndrome). The physician must avoid debating the validity, let alone the cure, of a given disease, and shift the focus onto function. Within that focus, attention to the patient's illness behaviors—his or her reactions to being sick—can be a therapeutic and limit-setting measure.[68] The patient's sick role identification must go beyond the privileges of the afflicted to include the complementary expectation that he or she will pursue health.[69]

REFERENCES

1. Bridges KW, Goldberg DP. Somatic presentation of DSM III psychiatric disorders in primary care. J Psychosom Res 1985;29:563–9.
2. Kroenke K, Price RK. Symptoms in the community. Prevalence, classification, and psychiatric comorbidity. Arch Intern Med 1993;153:2474–80.
3. Kroenke K, Spitzer RL, Williams JB. The PHQ-15: validity of a new measure for evaluating the severity of somatic symptoms. Psychosom Med 2002;64:258–66.
4. Kirmayer LJ, Robbins JM. Three forms of somatization in primary care: prevalence, co-occurrence, and sociodemographic characteristics. J Nerv Ment Dis 1991;179:647–55.
5. Gupta RK. Major depression: an illness with objective physical signs. World J Biol Psychiatry 2009;10:196–201.
6. Tylee A, Gandhi P. The importance of somatic symptoms in depression in primary care. Prim Care Companion J Clin Psychiatry 2005;7:167–76.
7. Nakao M, Yano E. Reporting of somatic symptoms as a screening marker for detecting major depression in a population of Japanese white-collar workers. J Clin Epidemiol 2003;56:1021–6.
8. Simon GE, VonKorff M, Piccinelli M, et al. An international study of the relation between somatic symptoms and depression. N Engl J Med 1999;341:1329–35.
9. Merskey H, Bogduk N, editors. Classification of chronic pain: descriptions of chronic pain syndromes and definition of pain terms. 2nd edition. Seattle (WA): IASP Press; 1994. p. 209–14.
10. Regier DA, Myers JK, Kramer M, et al. The NIMH epidemiologic catchment area program. Historical context, major objectives, and study population characteristics. Arch Gen Psychiatry 1984;41:934–41.
11. Breivik H, Collett B, Ventafridda V, et al. Survey of chronic pain in Europe: prevalence, impact on daily life, and treatment. Eur J Pain 2006;10:287–333.
12. Latham J, Davis BD. The socioeconomic impact of chronic pain. Disabil Rehabil 1994;16:39–44.

13. Breivik H, Borchgrevink PC, Allen SM, et al. Assessment of pain. Br J Anaesth 2008;101:17–24.
14. Ohayon MM, Schatzberg AF. Using chronic pain to predict depressive morbidity in the general population. Arch Gen Psychiatry 2003;60:39–47.
15. Bair MJ, Robinson RL, Katon W, et al. Depression and pain comorbidity: a literature review. Arch Intern Med 2003;163:2433–45.
16. Staiger TO, Gaster B, Sullivan MD, et al. Systematic review of antidepressants in the treatment of chronic low back pain. Spine 2003;28:2540–5.
17. Russell IJ, Mease PJ, Smith TR, et al. Efficacy and safety of duloxetine for treatment of fibromyalgia in patients with or without major depressive disorder: results from a 6-month, randomized, double-blind, placebo-controlled, fixed-dose trial. Pain 2008;136:432–44.
18. Max MB, Lynch SA, Muir J, et al. Effects of desipramine, amitriptyline, and fluoxetine on pain in diabetic neuropathy. N Engl J Med 1992;326:1250–6.
19. Kishore-Kumar R, Max MB, Schafer SC, et al. Desipramine relieves postherpetic neuralgia. Clin Pharmacol Ther 1990;47:305–12.
20. Smith TR. Duloxetine in diabetic neuropathy. Expert Opin Pharmacother 2006;7:215–23.
21. Arnold LM, Rosen A, Pritchett YL, et al. A randomized, double-blind, placebo-controlled trial of duloxetine in the treatment of women with fibromyalgia with or without major depressive disorder. Pain 2005;119:5–15.
22. Lang E, Liebig K, Kastner S, et al. Multidisciplinary rehabilitation versus usual care for chronic low back pain in the community: effects on quality of life. Spine J 2003;3:270–6.
23. Devine EC. Meta-analysis of the effect of psychoeducational interventions on pain in adults with cancer. Oncol Nurs Forum 2003;30:75–89.
24. Turk DC, Swanson KS, Tunks ER. Psychological approaches in the treatment of chronic pain patients—when pills, scalpels, and needles are not enough. Can J Psychiatry 2008;53:213–23.
25. Ohayon MM. Epidemiology of insomnia: what we know and what we still need to learn. Sleep Med Rev 2002;6:97–111.
26. Winkelman JW. Schizophrenia, obesity, and obstructive sleep apnea. J Clin Psychiatry 2001;62:8–11.
27. Ford DE, Kamerow DB. Epidemiologic study of sleep disturbances and psychiatric disorders. An opportunity for prevention? JAMA 1989;262:1479–84.
28. Buysse DJ, Reynolds CF 3rd, Kupfer DJ, et al. Clinical diagnoses in 216 insomnia patients using the International Classification of Sleep Disorders (ICSD), DSM-IV and ICD-10 categories: a report from the APA/NIMH DSM-IV Field Trial. Sleep 1994;17:630–7.
29. Mendlewicz J. Sleep disturbances: core symptoms of major depressive disorder rather than associated or comorbid disorders. World J Biol Psychiatry 2009;10:269–75.
30. Franzen PL, Buysse DJ. Sleep disturbances and depression: risk relationships for subsequent depression and therapeutic implications. Dialogues Clin Neurosci 2008;10:473–81.
31. Nierenberg AA, Husain MM, Trivedi MH, et al. Residual symptoms after remission of major depressive disorder with citalopram and risk of relapse: a STAR*D report. Psychol Med 2010;40:41–50.
32. Fava M. Pharmacological approaches to the treatment of residual symptoms. J Psychopharmacol 2006;20:29–34.

33. Ritterband LM, Thorndike FP, Gonder-Frederick LA, et al. Efficacy of an Internet-based behavioral intervention for adults with insomnia. Arch Gen Psychiatry 2009;66:692–8.

34. Sato M, Yamadera W, Matsushima M, et al. Clinical efficacy of individual cognitive behavior therapy for psychophysiological insomnia in 20 outpatients. Psychiatry Clin Neurosci 2010;64:187–95.

35. Wilson S, Argyropoulos S. Antidepressants and sleep: a qualitative review of the literature. Drugs 2005;65:927–47.

36. Mendelson WB. A review of the evidence for the efficacy and safety of trazodone in insomnia. J Clin Psychiatry 2005;66:469–76.

37. Wiegand MH. Antidepressants for the treatment of insomnia: a suitable approach? Drugs 2008;68:2411–7.

38. Asnis GM, Chakraburtty A, DuBoff EA, et al. Zolpidem for persistent insomnia in SSRI-treated depressed patients. J Clin Psychiatry 1999;60:668–76.

39. Fava M, McCall WV, Krystal A, et al. Eszopiclone co-administered with fluoxetine in patients with insomnia coexisting with major depressive disorder. Biol Psychiatry 2006;59:1052–60.

40. Fava M, Thase ME, DeBattista C. A multicenter, placebo-controlled study of modafinil augmentation in partial responders to selective serotonin reuptake inhibitors with persistent fatigue and sleepiness. J Clin Psychiatry 2005;66:85–93.

41. Frye MA, Grunze H, Suppes T, et al. A placebo-controlled evaluation of adjunctive modafinil in the treatment of bipolar depression. Am J Psychiatry 2007;164:1242–9.

42. Parker G, Brotchie H. Do the old psychostimulant drugs have a role in managing treatment-resistant depression? Acta Psychiatr Scand 2010;121(4):308–14.

43. Chapman IM. The anorexia of aging. Clin Geriatr Med 2007;23:735–56, v.

44. Klein KM, Theisen F, Knake S, et al. Topiramate, nutrition, and weight change: a prospective study. J Neurol Neurosurg Psychiatry 2008;79:590–3.

45. Laimer M, Kramer-Reinstadler K, Rauchenzauner M, et al. Effect of mirtazapine treatment on body composition and metabolism. J Clin Psychiatry 2006;67:421–4.

46. Riechelmann RP, Burman D, Tannock IF, et al. Phase II trial of mirtazapine for cancer-related cachexia and anorexia. Am J Hosp Palliat Care 2010;27:106–10.

47. Gartlehner G, Thieda P, Hansen RA, et al. Comparative risk for harms of second-generation antidepressants: a systematic review and meta-analysis. Drug Saf 2008;31:851–65.

48. World Health Organization. ICD-10: international statistical classification of diseases and related health problems. 10th revision. Geneva (Switzerland): World Health Organization; 1992.

49. Harvey SB, Wessely S, Kuh D, et al. The relationship between fatigue and psychiatric disorders: evidence for the concept of neurasthenia. J Psychosom Res 2009;66:445–54.

50. Ridsdale L, Evans A, Jerrett W, et al. Patients who consult with tiredness: frequency of consultation, perceived causes of tiredness and its association with psychological distress. Br J Gen Pract 1994;44:413–6.

51. Bell CM, Fischer HD, Gill SS, et al. Initiation of benzodiazepines in the elderly after hospitalization. J Gen Intern Med 2007;22:1024–9.

52. Barton C, Sklenicka J, Sayegh P, et al. Contraindicated medication use among patients in a memory disorders clinic. Am J Geriatr Pharmacother 2008;6:147–52.

53. Laumann EO, Paik A, Rosen RC. Sexual dysfunction in the United States: prevalence and predictors. JAMA 1999;281:537–44.
54. Kennedy SH, Rizvi S. Sexual dysfunction, depression, and the impact of antidepressants. J Clin Psychopharmacol 2009;29:157–64.
55. Schweitzer I, Maguire K, Ng C. Sexual side-effects of contemporary antidepressants: review. Aust N Z J Psychiatry 2009;43:795–808.
56. Kennedy SH, Dickens SE, Eisfeld BS, et al. Sexual dysfunction before antidepressant therapy in major depression. J Affect Disord 1999;56:201–8.
57. Araujo AB, Durante R, Feldman HA, et al. The relationship between depressive symptoms and male erectile dysfunction: cross-sectional results from the Massachusetts male aging study. Psychosom Med 1998;60:458–65.
58. Rosen RC, Seidman SN, Menza MA, et al. Quality of life, mood, and sexual function: a path analytic model of treatment effects in men with erectile dysfunction and depressive symptoms. Int J Impot Res 2004;16:334–40.
59. Saiz-Ruiz J, Montes JM, Ibanez A, et al. Assessment of sexual functioning in depressed patients treated with mirtazapine: a naturalistic 6-month study. Hum Psychopharmacol 2005;20:435–40.
60. Perlis RH, Fava M, Nierenberg AA, et al. Strategies for treatment of SSRI-associated sexual dysfunction: a survey of an academic psychopharmacology practice. Harv Rev Psychiatry 2002;10:109–14.
61. Seidman SN, Roose SP, Menza MA, et al. Treatment of erectile dysfunction in men with depressive symptoms: results of a placebo-controlled trial with sildenafil citrate. Am J Psychiatry 2001;158:1623–30.
62. Fava M, Nurnberg HG, Seidman SN, et al. Efficacy and safety of sildenafil in men with serotonergic antidepressant-associated erectile dysfunction: results from a randomized, double-blind, placebo-controlled trial. J Clin Psychiatry 2006;67:240–6.
63. Nurnberg HG, Hensley PL, Heiman JR, et al. Sildenafil treatment of women with antidepressant-associated sexual dysfunction: a randomized controlled trial. JAMA 2008;300:395–404.
64. Huynh NN, McIntyre RS. What are the implications of the STAR*D trial for primary care? a review and synthesis. Prim Care Companion J Clin Psychiatry 2008;10:91–6.
65. Kontos N, Freudenreich O, Querques J. Ownership, responsibility and hospital care: Lessons for the consultation psychiatrist. Gen Hosp Psychiatry 2008;30:257–62.
66. Kroenke K, Jackson JL, Chamberlin J. Depressive and anxiety disorders in patients presenting with physical complaints: clinical predictors and outcome. Am J Med 1997;103:339–47.
67. Smith GR Jr, Rost K, Kashner TM. A trial of the effect of a standardized psychiatric consultation on health outcomes and costs in somatizing patients. Arch Gen Psychiatry 1995;52:238–43.
68. Mechanic D. Sociological dimensions of illness behavior. Soc Sci Med 1995;41:1207–16.
69. Parsons T. The social system. New York: The Free Press; 1951.

An Approach to Selected Legal Issues: Confidentiality, Mandatory Reporting, Abuse and Neglect, Informed Consent, Capacity Decisions, Boundary Issues, and Malpractice Claims

Rebecca Weintraub Brendel, MD, JD[a,b,*],
Marlynn H. Wei, MD, JD[a,b], Ronald Schouten, MD, JD[a,b],
Judith G. Edersheim, JD, MD[a,b]

KEYWORDS

- Medicolegal issues • Malpractice • Informed consent
- Reporting obligations

Medical practice occurs within a legal and regulatory context. This article covers several of the legal issues that frequently arise in the general medical setting. While this article provides an overview of approaches to informed consent, boundary issues, and malpractice claims, it is critical for clinicians to be familiar with the specific requirements and standards in the jurisdictions in which they practice. As a general rule, it is most important that physicians recognize that the best way to avoid legal problems is to be aware of legal requirements in the jurisdictions in which they practice, but to think clinically and not legally in the provision of consistent and sound clinical care to their patients.[1]

[a] Department of Psychiatry, Massachusetts General Hospital, 15 Parkman Street, WAC 812, Boston, MA 02114, USA
[b] Department of Psychiatry, Harvard Medical School, 25 Shattuck Street, Boston, MA 02115, USA
* Corresponding author. Department of Psychiatry, Massachusetts General Hospital, 15 Parkman Street, WAC 812, Boston, MA 02114.
E-mail address: rbrendel@partners.org

Med Clin N Am 94 (2010) 1229–1240
doi:10.1016/j.mcna.2010.08.003
0025-7125/10/$ – see front matter © 2010 Elsevier Inc. All rights reserved.

medical.theclinics.com

CONFIDENTIALITY AND MANDATORY REPORTING LAWS

Confidentiality has been a central feature of the physician-patient relationship for centuries. As early as 430 BC, confidentiality was codified in the Hippocratic Oath, "Whatever I see or hear, professionally or privately, which ought not to be divulged, I will keep secret and tell no one."[2] The principle of confidentiality remains an important ethical, legal, and professional practice in clinical medicine.[3,4] The absolute confidentiality of the Hippocratic Oath, however, has given way to several exceptions that reflect a complex balance between the importance of privacy as a necessary component of the doctor-patient relationship that respects patient autonomy and facilitates honest information-sharing for treatment on the one hand, and the many demands of an ever more complex society on the other. Specifically, courts and legislatures have determined that certain concerns, such as public safety, justify modification of absolute confidentiality.

Examples of situations in which public policy considerations limit doctor-patient confidentiality include mandated reporting of infectious diseases and suspected child and elder abuse. States and the federal government have regulations that govern which communicable diseases should be reported to local and state authorities and/or the Centers for Disease Control and Prevention (CDC); this list is revised annually.[5]

State law governs mandated reporting of infectious diseases; thus reportable diseases vary from jurisdiction to jurisdiction. Physicians should be aware of which diseases are reportable in the jurisdictions in which they practice and what information must be reported, along with the positive test results. That being said, all states require reporting of internationally quarantinable diseases (including cholera, plague, and yellow fever) in compliance with the World Health Organization's International Health Regulations.[6] States may also have different requirements for what information must be reported along with a positive test result for a communicable disease. For example, although a majority of states require confidential name-based reporting of adolescents and adults who test positive for human immunodeficiency virus (HIV) infection, states nonetheless may employ different requirements for reporting of positive HIV tests, varying from anonymized or de-identified reporting to confidential identified reporting.[7] In addition, state law varies regarding whether written permission is required to release information about HIV test results and whether partner/spousal notification is mandatory.[7] Regardless of the state requirements for HIV-reporting, since the emergence of the AIDS epidemic in the early 1980s, states have adopted AIDS reporting practices that ultimately culminate in the relay of de-identified information to the CDC for the purpose of national surveillance.[7]

The emergence of policy that is related to infectious disease reporting for the purpose of public health has led to additional exceptions to confidentiality for public safety and welfare considerations. One such area includes the duty to warn or protect third parties from, threatened physical harm from a patient. This type of duty was established in the landmark 1976 California court decision of *Tarasoff v Board of Regents*.[8,9] This case established that under California law, clinicians could have an obligation to a third party or parties (ie, an individual or individuals outside of the doctor-patient relationship or second-party relationship) in certain circumstances in which the patient posed a risk of harm to that party. In reaching this decision, the court drew, in part, on infectious disease-related exceptions to confidentiality, to support a balancing of patients' rights to privacy against public interest. Specifically, the Court held that "the public interest in supporting effective treatment of mental illness and in protecting the rights of patients to privacy ... must be weighed against the public interest in safety from violent assault."[9]

In the area of the duty to protect, it is especially critical for practitioners to be aware of the legal requirements in the jurisdictions in which they practice because of variations in whether a duty exists, to whom the duty applies, what set of circumstances triggers the duty, and what actions discharge the physician's obligation. For example, although a majority of states have passed laws that require licensed mental health professionals to disclose a dangerous patient's confidential communications for the purposes of protecting potential victims when a patient poses a serious threat of harm to another person,[10,11] a small minority of states have rejected the duty to warn/protect and still others may rely on judicial opinions (common law) for the characteristics of the duty. In addition, duty to warn/protect laws may not cover all members of a treatment team. Specifically, some states, such as Massachusetts, apply the duty to psychiatric physicians and licensed mental health professionals but not to other physicians.[1] In Massachusetts, as in many other states, where a duty to protect exists, it may be discharged by taking steps to protect the potential victim by voluntary hospitalization of the patient, taking steps toward involuntary hospitalizations, or warning the victim or law enforcement. Preference is given to steps that violate confidentiality to the least extent possible while still protecting the potential victims(s).

In states with statutes that govern the duty to warn/protect, the scope of the duty is generally limited to situations in which there is a specific threat to an identifiable third party, circumstances in which the patient has a known history of violence, and/or cases in which there is a reasonable reason to anticipate violence. As noted, state laws may also outline measures (including notifying law enforcement, hospitalizing the patient, or warning the potential victim) that may be taken to discharge the duty to warn.[12]

ABUSE AND NEGLECT

Unlike the varying state laws on the duty to warn/protect third parties, physicians across the United States are under clear obligation to report child and elder abuse and neglect to state authorities.[13,14] Federal law sets the minimum standard for what actions and/or failures to act constitute child abuse and neglect, and state legislatures vary in terms of the definition of child abuse.[14] States generally define child abuse as "harm or substantial risk of harm" or "serious threat or serious harm" to a person younger than 18 years.[14]

Elder abuse and neglect similarly varies among jurisdictions. However, in general, most states include 5 elements: infliction of pain or injury, infliction of emotional or psychological harm, sexual assault, material or financial exploitation, and neglect.[15] In the context of elder neglect, the report may arise from self-neglect. Physicians are considered mandated reporters and should therefore be familiar with the reporting requirements and available screening and investigative resources and agencies in their jurisdiction. The underreporting and underdetection of elder abuse remains problematic.[16]

While most physicians are often concerned that reporting abuse and neglect to state agencies may constitute a breach of confidentiality and result in liability, they should be aware that failure to report abuse and neglect is more likely to create liability than is making a mandated report. Specifically, states may impose liability for failure to make a mandated report, and physicians may be liable under civil law for downstream harm to a child if the failure to report was negligent or below the standard of care. In addition, good-faith reporting in reliance on the law is a valid defense to a claim of breach of confidentiality brought against the physician. Most jurisdictions apply a reasonable suspicion standard such that reporting providers are not required to have definitive proof or evidence of abuse or neglect, but should exercise professional judgment and good faith in making a report of suspected abuse or neglect.[13,15] In other words, absent intentional misconduct, so long as the physician can substantiate the report with the reasons for which child abuse or neglect is suspected and can demonstrate a reasonable thought process in making the report, the physician would not face liability for making a report, even if the allegations of abuse/neglect prove unsubstantiated on further investigation.

OTHER REPORTING OBLIGATIONS

Depending on one's jurisdiction, physicians have varying obligations to report certain types of injuries, gunshot wounds, and injuries resulting from some forms of criminal behavior to local authorities.[17,18] These exceptions to confidentiality, like the examples given above, stem from public safety and welfare considerations. First, burn injuries are generally reportable to local authorities; however, the reporting obligations differ regarding the cause of the burn, the degree of the burn, and the extent of the burn. For example, gunshot wound laws often cover powder burns as distinct from other types of burns.[19,20] Some states require reporting of all second- and third-degree burns, and others require reporting of burns that cover a certain percentage of body surface area (eg, 5% or more in Massachusetts).[17] State law definitions of reportable burns may also include inhalation burns and injuries caused by fireworks.[21]

Reporting of gunshot wounds may require physicians to report a gunshot wound[22] and also a powder burn, bullet hole, or other injuring caused by the discharge of a firearm.[19,23] Other life-threatening wounds may also be reportable, although there are sometimes exceptions if the injury was clearly the result of nonintentional actions or an accident.[24] These wounds, for example, could include stab wounds or wounds by a knife or other sharp, pointed instrument.[19,24,25]

Mandated reporting for sexual assault is limited to those that would qualify under child abuse.[26] A small minority of states requires reporting of domestic violence, even when the victim is a competent adult.[27] Although very few states have explicit domestic violence reporting statutes, laws that mandate reporting of nonaccidental or intentionally inflicted serious injuries or serious injuries that result from illegal or criminal conduct may also cover domestic violence–related injuries.[28] Unlike mandated reporting of suspected abuse and neglect, communicable diseases, and the duty to warn/protect, physicians may face criminal liability for failure to make a mandated report of a gunshot-related wound or other injury related to violent or criminal activity. In general, states that impose criminal liability for failure to make these reports limit criminal liability to a misdemeanor, but it is important to be aware that punishment can include incarceration for up to 1 year.[22]

HEALTH INSURANCE PORTABILITY AND ACCOUNTABILITY ACT

As the preceding sections have illustrated, absolute doctor-patient confidentiality has given way to several exceptions based on public health, welfare, and safety rationales. As the American health care system has become increasingly complex, administrative simplification and efficiency of health care delivery have also become rationales for limiting confidentiality. Specifically, the Health Insurance Portability and Accountability Act (HIPAA) was enacted by the US Congress in 1996 and raised concerns at the time within the medical community about its impact on how confidential patient information was handled.[29–31] HIPAA is federal legislation that governs the management of "protected health information," which includes information that identifies a patient (such as demographic data), that concerns a mental or physical condition, and describes services or treatment provided or relates to payment.[32] HIPAA covers disclosure of medical information, patient access to information, and a new category of record established under HIPAA called "psychotherapy notes." Contrary to increasing the privacy of medical records, HIPAA increased the circumstances under which protected health information could be released without specific consent from a patient.[30]

Legislators intended HIPAA to improve the efficiency and effectiveness of the health care system. The privacy rule categorized what information is considered protected information so as to protect confidentiality and privacy, but also recognized the modernization and trend toward electronic medical records and the need for entities to share these records.[30] HIPAA allows covered entities to release protected health information for the purposes of treatment, payment, and health care operations without specific authorization or consent by the patient.[30] However, HIPAA limits disclosure by requiring covered entities to follow the "minimum necessary" principle, stating that the covered entity must use reasonable efforts to disclose and request only the minimum amount of protected health information needed to accomplish the intended purpose of the use, disclosure, or request.[33] Therefore, clinicians should use critical judgment in determining what information needs to be disclosed. Furthermore, hospitals must inform patients of the institution's practices under HIPAA in the form of privacy notices. Patients may also request records of disclosures of their protected health information. Finally, federal and state laws with stricter protections of specific health information preempt HIPAA. Therefore, written consent may still be required for its release under additional federal and state regulations, including information such as HIV status and treatment, genetic testing, records relating to alcohol and substance abuse treatment programs, and domestic violence and sexual assault records.[18] Of note, HIPAA does not prevent the release of information in emergency settings or settings in which there are mandated reporting obligations. As a general rule, all records, medical and psychiatric, in the patient's medical chart are accessible by the patient. Patients may be denied access to their records only in narrow circumstances, where a licensed professional reasonably finds that the record would harm, endanger the life of, or jeopardize the physical safety of the patient or another person.[18]

As a general rule, however, physicians should approach situations from their duty to confidentiality, and any breaches should be carefully considered. Clinicians should always limit the amount of information disclosed to the minimum necessary, and consider other available alternatives to avoid necessitating a breach of confidentiality before releasing information to a third party.

TREATMENT: CONSENT AND REFUSAL

Any unauthorized and unjustified touching, including contact for medical interventions, is considered battery under civil law. Thus, a patient must give informed consent for any medical intervention.[34] The doctrine of informed consent emerged from the period of extending patients' right to self-determination.[35] Informed consent gave patients the right to choose how they would be treated.[35] Informed consent is the process by which the patient determines whether to accept or refuse the treatment offered by a physician or another clinician. The focus is not on the written consent form but on the process of communication, information exchange, and acceptance or rejection of the medical intervention.[36]

The threshold determination for informed consent is decisional capacity. Capacity determines whether patients have the ability to consent to or refuse medical treatment. Psychiatrists are often asked to assess the quality of the patient's decision-making process, often when the patient refuses a medical intervention recommended by treating physicians. The assessment of decision-making ability is a clinical determination of an individual's ability to perform a task or to execute a set of functions, and it can be performed by any physician with the requisite knowledge and experience.[37] The legal equivalent of capacity is competency, which requires a judicial determination. Under the law, all adults are presumed competent. Competency may be global in certain cases (such as the case of a patient in a coma). However, capacity and competency must be evaluated in the context of a specific task. Different tasks require different abilities, information, and thresholds of understanding. Therefore, the initial inquiry for a capacity evaluation is the question, "Capacity for what?" The clinician can then use this information, including whether the patient has been presented with the decision and whether he or she is accepting or refusing a recommended procedure, to determine the elements of a capacity assessment.

CAPACITY DECISIONS

Over the past 4 decades, a practical framework for the assessment of decisional capacity for medical decisions has emerged.[38–40] For a person to possess decisional capacity, 4 conditions must be met.[41] First, the person must be able to express a consistent preference. A person who cannot or is unwilling to express a preference presumptively lacks capacity. Second, the individual must understand the facts surrounding the decisions being made. The treating physicians should educate the patient about the proposed treatment, including its risks and benefits. The patient must be able to retain the information when it is presented and to use it appropriately in decision-making. Third, the person must be able to express an appreciation of how the facts pertain to him or her, including the risks and benefits of action versus nonaction. Lastly, the individual must be able to rationally manipulate data in the decision-making process. The rational manipulation requirement is assessed in view of the person's life and circumstances, including previous behavior and guiding principles (eg, religion and culture, and past choices).[41]

INFORMED CONSENT

In addition to decisional capacity, informed consent requires that the patient's decision be knowing (or intelligent) and voluntary.[32,42–45] Physicians owe their patients a fiduciary duty, and this duty includes an obligation to act in the patient's interests by disclosing all information material to those interests.[46] The standard for determining how to assess what information a physician must share with a patient to meet the knowing prong of informed consent varies. In a small majority of states, the legal standard for disclosure to patients is that which a "reasonable medical practitioner" would provide. The advantage of this standard is that it is practical and knowable for a physician to determine what the practices of the medical community are. On the other hand, a minority of states employ the "reasonable patient standard," which focuses on what the reasonable patient would want to know. In these states, the clinician is required to provide the amount of information that would be used by a reasonable or average patient in making an informed decision. Some states take the patient-based standard even further, employing a materiality standard that requires the physician to include information that would be relevant to the particular patient.[1] Requirements for information that must be disclosed vary among states, and may include reasonably foreseeable risks of treatment and alternative available treatments.[44] Litigation may arise from disputes over the physicians' duty to disclose all reasonably foreseeable risks, duty to disclose alternatives, and causation of injury.[44]

Although the standard for information varies among jurisdictions, as a general rule of thumb for clinical practice and risk management, providing more information reduces the risk of litigation. Overall, regardless of jurisdiction, clinicians will generally meet the standard for providing adequate information if they share 6 broad categories of information with their patient:

1. The diagnosis and the nature of the condition being treated
2. The reasonably expected benefits from the proposed treatment
3. The nature and likelihood of the risks involved
4. The inability to precisely predict results of the treatment
5. The potential irreversibility of the treatment
6. The expected risks, benefits, and results of alternative, or no, treatment.[47]

The process should be an open discussion and exchange of information between the doctor and the patient.[47]

The voluntariness of informed consent requires that consent be obtained without coercion, and without external forces that limit the autonomy of the patient.[34] The assessment of voluntariness is complex, including, for example, questions of whether individuals are pressured by family members.[48] One particular area where voluntariness may be at particular issue is in the case of institutionalized or incarcerated individuals who may not perceive that they have the right to or the option of refusing an intervention.

Informed consent is not required for initiation of treatment in certain situations, most commonly for emergency treatment.[49] Emergency treatments are those in which the failure to treat would result in serious and potentially irreversible deterioration of a patient's condition. Treatment under this exception can only be continued until the patient is stabilized. If the physician has knowledge that a patient would have refused the emergency intervention, when competent the patient's prior expressed decision cannot be overridden. Other exceptions where informed consent is not required include waiver and therapeutic privilege.[49] Patients may waive consent and choose to defer to the judgment of the clinician or to another individual; the capacity to waive consent should be documented. Therapeutic privilege applies where physicians determine that the consent process itself would contribute to the worsening of a patient's condition; in such a situation consent should be obtained from another decision-maker. However, therapeutic privilege does not apply if the concern is that the consent process would make the patient less likely to accept treatment. However, both of these exceptions should be applied narrowly and only in specific circumstances.

ADVANCED DIRECTIVES AND SURROGATE DECISION MAKING

If a patient lacks capacity, and therefore the ability to provide informed consent or refusal for treatment, a substituted decision-maker is required to make decisions regarding medical intervention or nonintervention. Substitute decision-makers are required to assess and decide based on what the patient would have wanted had the patient been able to make his or her own decisions; this is also known as the substitute judgment standard. In some cases, the decision-maker may be asked to make decisions based on the patient's best interest.

Substituted decision-makers are appointed through multiple avenues and include informal mechanisms (eg, advance directives, surrogate decision-making statutes) and the formal, court-ordered mechanism of guardianships. Advance directives include the health care proxy and durable power of attorney, both of which contain a "springing clause." These documents, once executed, do not take effect until the patient is deemed to lack decision-making ability, and state law generally requires documentation of decisional incapacity by a physician to invoke the powers of the surrogate decision-maker. The advance directive then continues in effect until such time as a patient regains decisional capacity. Many individuals still do not have advance directives and, in the absence of an advance directive, some states have statutory provisions on how to appoint substitute decision-makers (eg, ranking priorities among guardians, spouses, or adult children).[50] In addition, some jurisdictions have state statutes and case law that create a formal mechanism for guardianship or court approval for medical decision-making.[51]

The appointment of a guardian is typically motivated by concerns that arise when a patient is unable to make medical decisions in the absence of an advance directive. Guardianship is the "delegation, by the state, of authority over an individual's person or estate to another party."[52] Guardianship statutes vary from state to state, and courts review these petitions for guardianship under the standard of incompetency outlined in state statutes.[53] Evolving legal standards for guardianship support limited guardianships that delegate authority only for the specific decisions and functions that an individual is unable to perform (thereby retaining as much of the individual's autonomy and right to self-determination as possible).

MALPRACTICE

Physicians owe a duty of care to their patients, ethically and legally. Legal liability is a source of concern for many physicians, leading some to practice so-called defensive medicine, characterized by making decisions based in part or in whole on the desire to avoid legal liability. While physicians should be aware of the requirements of competent care and understand the foundation of malpractice liability, overreliance on the law and on excessive measures to avoid liability should be placed aside in favor of sound clinical judgment and practice as a means of avoiding liability.

A claim of malpractice is based on 4 elements, often referred to as the "4 Ds." To make a successful claim, the patient or plaintiff must establish that a Duty or doctor-patient relationship existed, that there was a Dereliction, or breach, of the duty, that the breach of the duty caused Direct harm to the patient, and that the breach of the duty caused Damages. Some physicians and commentators worry that malpractice awards do not reflect compensation for negligently-inflicted injuries, but rather an insurance policy for any bad outcome, regardless of negligence. In addition, attention has focused on the emergence of a national crisis related to skyrocketing awards and escalating premiums.

In reality, only a small number of cases involving injury due to medical errors result in litigation, and defendants prevail in the majority of malpractice litigations. In addition, the median malpractice award has been essentially flat for a decade and, while increasing premiums are related to the size of awards, there are also data to suggest that premium increases are related to stock market performance and have not outpaced other practice expenses. Nevertheless, malpractice awards do occur in the absence of negligence, and being sued for malpractice is associated with personal and professional stress, regardless of the outcome.

Several factors are associated with malpractice risk reduction. First, because physicians with poor communication skills are at increased risk of being sued, improving communication between physician and patient is a key element of risk reduction. Second, acknowledging error and preserving the doctor-patient relationship are other factors associated with a reduction of the risk of malpractice litigation. In light of this, many states have enacted laws to facilitate disclosure of errors and open discussion of adverse outcomes. These "apology laws" promote honest communication and disclosure of unexpected adverse outcomes by excluding physician apologies (and in some states other information shared in the course of an apology) from evidence of fault should malpractice litigation ensue.[54]

Other factors associated with malpractice risk reduction include recognition of individual and systemic factors that contribute to errors, maintenance of good clinical records, consultation with colleagues, and avoidance of "overlegalization" of clinical practice. Although physicians should be aware of applicable laws in the jurisdiction in which they practice, the best method to avoid liability is through the provision of sound clinical care.

One specific area that may lead to professional liability is that of boundary violations, or behaviors that involve an inappropriate departure from the accepted doctor and patient roles, as defined by societal and professional standards.[55] Boundary violations are the departure from the fiduciary duty of the physician to act only in the patient's interest, rather than in the physician's interest.[55] Boundary violations may take many forms including, but not limited to, taking financial advantage of a patient, using the doctor-patient contact to gratify the practitioner's own needs, and sexual activity with patients.

Self-reported physician boundary violations of patients have an estimated prevalence of between 3.3% and 14.5%.[56] Studies indicate that disciplinary actions by state medical boards and federal agencies for sex-related offenses are brought against 0.02% to 1.6% of physicians. Heightened risk of sexual boundary violations have been found in the specialties of family medicine, psychiatry, and obstetrics/gynecology. The majority of sexual boundary offenders are male.[56] Although ethical decisions about boundary violations are guided by ethics codes from professional organizations, these groups are voluntary membership organizations and cannot take disciplinary action against nonmembers. However, the codes of these organizations may be relied on by courts and by licensure boards as evidence of the professional standard of care and practice, and it is therefore important for physicians to be aware of the ethical tenets of the major organizations in their field of practice, even if they are nonmembers.[57] Of particular note, the American Medical Association (AMA) position on sexual misconduct is clear; it defines any sexual contact concurrent with the patient-physician relationship as misconduct.[58] In addition, the AMA position considers sexual or romantic relationships with former patients unethical if the physician exploits trust or knowledge from the previous professional relationship.

SUMMARY

Medical practice occurs amidst a complex legal and regulatory framework. Major areas of law related to clinical practice include confidentiality and exceptions to confidentiality, informed consent and treatment refusal, and malpractice. Physicians should be aware of the relevant standards and requirements in the jurisdiction(s) in which they practice but, to reduce liability and to provide sound clinical care, should avoid overreliance on the law and overlegalization of the doctor-patient relationship in favor of open and effective communication with patients, sound clinical judgment, consultation with colleagues to promote effective care, and attention paid to recognizing and ameliorating individual and systemic factors that contribute to error. These goals also require that physicians maintain proper boundaries with their patients in accordance with legal, regulatory, and ethical principles.

REFERENCES

1. Schouten R, Brendel RW. Common pitfalls in giving medical-legal advice to trainees and supervisees. Harv Rev Psychiatry 2009;17(4):291–4.
2. Chadwick J, Mann WN. Hippocrates. The Oath. In: Lloyd GER, editor. Hippocratic writings. London: Penguin Books; 1983. p. 67.

3. American Medical Association. Opinion 5.05: confidentiality. Available at: http://www.ama-assn.org/ama/pub/physician-resources/medical-ethics/code-medical-ethics/opinion505.shtml. Accessed March 21, 2010.

4. American Psychiatric Association. Position statement on confidentiality. Washington, DC: American Psychiatric Association; 1978.

5. Centers for Disease Control and Prevention. Nationally notifiable conditions. Available at: http://www.cdc.gov/ncphi/disss/nndss/phs/infdis.htm. Accessed March 21, 2010.

6. Centers for Disease Control and Prevention. National notifiable diseases surveillance system. Available at: http://www.cdc.gov/ncphi/disss/nndss/nndsshis.htm. Accessed on March 21, 2010.

7. Brendel RW, Cohen MA. Ethical issues, advance directives, and surrogate decision-making. In: Cohen MA, Gorman J, editors. Comprehensive textbook of AIDS psychiatry. New York: Oxford University Press; 2008. p. 577–84.

8. Schuck PH, Givelber DJ. Tarasoff v Regents of the University of California: the therapist's dilemma. In: Rabin RL, Sugarman SD, editors. Tort stories. New York: Foundation Press; 2003. p. 99–128.

9. *Tarasoff v Board of Regents of the University of California*, 17 Cal. 3d425, 551 P.2d 334, 131 Cal. Rptr. 14 (Cal 1976).

10. Harris GC. The dangerous patient exception to the psychotherapist-patient privilege: the Tarasoff Duty and the Jaffee Footnote. Wash Law Rev 1999;74:33–46.

11. Klinka E. It's been a privilege: advising patients of the Tarasoff Duty and its legal consequences for the Federal psychotherapist-patient privilege. Fordham Law Rev 2009;78:863.

12. Duty to warn patient's potential victims; cause of action 2005, 123 Ch. § 36B; Mass. Gen. Laws.

13. Schouten R. Legal responsibilities with child abuse and domestic violence. In: Jacobson JL, Jacobson AM, editors. Psychiatric secrets. Philadelphia: Hanley & Belfus; 2001.

14. Milosavljevic N, Brendel RW. Abuse and neglect. In: Stern TA, Rosenbaum JF, Fava M, et al, editors. Comprehensive clinical psychiatry. Philadelphia: Mosby/Elsevier; 2008. p. 1133–42.

15. Kazim A, Brendel RW. Abuse and neglect. In: Stern TA, Herman JB, editors. Massachusetts general hospital psychiatry update and board preparation. 2nd edition. New York: McGraw-Hill; 2004. p. 539–44.

16. Kahan FS, Paris BE. Why elder abuse continues to elude the health care system. Mt Sinai J Med 2003;70:62–8.

17. Houry D, Sachs CJ, Feldhaus KM, et al. Violence-inflicted injuries: reporting laws in the fifty states. Ann Emerg Med 2002;39(1):56–60.

18. Frampton A. Reporting of gunshot wounds by doctors in emergency departments: a duty or a right? Some legal and ethical issues surrounding breaking patient confidentiality. Emerg Med J 2005;22:84–6.

19. Massachusetts General Laws, Ch. 112, S. 12a.

20. Kansas Statute 2006, §21–4213.

21. Conn. General Statute Sec 2003. 19a–510a.

22. Texas Health and Safety Code Ann. S 2007. § 161.041.

23. New York CLS Penal 2010. § 265.25.

24. N.C. Gen. Stat. 2007. § 90–21.20

25. Hawaii Rev Stat. 453–14. Available at: http://www.capitol.hawaii.gov/hrscurrent/Vol10_Ch0436-0474/HRS0453/HRS_0453-0014.htm. Accessed August 10, 2010.

26. National District Attorneys Organization, Mandatory reporting of child abuse and neglect: state statutes and professional ethics. Available at: http://www.ndaa.org/pdf/mandatory_reporting_state_statutes.pdf. Accessed August 10, 2010.
27. National Center for the Prosecution of Violence Against Women, APRI, summary of laws relevant to the mandatory reporting of domestic violence when the victim is a competent adult. Available at: http://www.ndaa.org/pdf/dv_summary.pdf; 2006. Accessed August 10, 2010.
28. Hyman A, Schillinger D, Lo B. Laws mandating reporting of domestic violence—do they promote well-being? JAMA 1995;273(22):1781–4.
29. Health Insurance Portability and Accountability Act of 1996. Public Law 1996:104–91.
30. Brendel RW, Bryan E. HIPAA for psychiatrists. Harv Rev Psychiatry 2004;12: 177–83.
31. Health Insurance Portablity and Accountability Act (HIPAA): its broad effect on practice. Am J Gastroenterol 2005;100:1440–3.
32. HIPAA Privacy Rule. 45, 164.512. 2001. C.F.R.
33. HIPAA Privacy Rule. 45, 164.502(b), 164.514(d). 2001. C.F.R.
34. Appelbaum PS, Lidz CW, Meisel A. Informed consent: legal theory and clinical practice. New York: Oxford University Press; 1987.
35. Katz J. The silent world of doctor and patient. New York: Free Press; 1984. 48–9.
36. Schouten R, Edersheim JG. Informed consent, competency, treatment refusal, and civil commitment. In: Stern TA, Rosenbaum JF, Fava M, et al, editors. Massachusetts General Hospital comprehensive clinical psychiatry. Philadelphia: Mosby/Elsevier; 2008. p. 1143–54.
37. Appelbaum PS, Roth LH. Clinical issues in the assessment of competency. Am J Psychiatry 1981;138:1462–7.
38. Appelbaum PS, Grisso T. Assessing patients' capacities to consent to treatment. N Engl J Med 1988;319:1635–8.
39. Meisel A, Rotrh LH, Lidz CW. Toward a model of legal doctrine of informed consent. Am J Psychiatry 1977;134:285–9.
40. Roth LH, Meisel A, LIdz CW. Tests of competency to consent to treatment. Am J Psychiatry 1977;134:279–84.
41. Appelbaum PS. Assessment of patients' competence to consent to treatment. N Engl J Med 2007;357:1834–7.
42. Schloendorff v Society of New York Hospital, 92 105, NE (1914).
43. Salgo v Leland Stanford, Jr. University Board of Trustees, 170 P2d 317, 170–182 (Cal Court of Appeals 1957).
44. Natanson v Kline, 1093 P2nd 350, 1093–1109 (1960) Supreme Court of Kansas.
45. Canterbury v Spence, 772 F2.d 464, (DC Cir. cert. denied, 409 U.S. 1064).
46. Schuck PH. Rethinking informed consent. Yale Law J 1994;103:899–959.
47. King JS, Moulton BW. Rethinking informed consent: the case for shared medical decision-making. Am J Law Med 2006;32:429–93.
48. Roberts LW. Informed consent and the capacity for voluntarism. Am J Psychiatry 2002;159:705–12.
49. Meisel A. The "exceptions" to the informed consent doctrine: striking a balance between competing value in medical decision making. Wis L Rev 1979;413–88.
50. Health Care Surrogate Act of 2005, 755, 40. Ill. Comp. Stat.
51. Ch. 201, § 1–15 (2009); Mass. Gen. Laws.

52. Melton GB, Petrila J, Poythress NG, et al. Psychological evaluations for the courts: a handbook for mental health professionals and lawyers. 2nd edition. New York: Guilford Press; 1997. p. 339.

53. Karp N, Wood E. Guardianship monitoring: a national survey of court practices. Available at: www.guardianship.org/reports/07GuardianshipMonitoring.pdf; 2006. Accessed August 10, 2010.

54. Gallagher TH, Studdert D, Levinson W. Disclosing harmful medical errors to patients. N Engl J Med 2007;2713–9.

55. Schouten R, Brendel RW, Edersheim JG. Malpractice and boundary violations. In: Stern TA, Rosenbaum JF, Fava M, et al, editors. Massachusetts General Hospital comprehensive clinical psychiatry. Philadelphia: Mosby/Elsevier; 2008. p. 1165–75.

56. Sansone RA, Sansone LA. Crossing the line: sexual boundary violations by physicians. Psychiatry 2009;6(6):45–8.

57. Benedek EP, Wahl D. Sexual misconduct, The American Psychiatric Association, and the American Medical Association. In: Bloom JD, editor. Physician sexual misconduct. Washington, DC: American Psychiatric Press; 1999. p. 91–107.

58. American Medical Association, Opinion 8.14 Sexual misconduct in the practice of medicine. AMA Code of Medical Ethics. Available at: http://www.ama-assn.org/ama/pub/physician-resources/medical-ethics/code-medical-ethics/opinion814.shtml. Accessed February 19, 2010.

An Approach to the Patient with Organ Failure: Transplantation and End-of-Life Treatment Decisions

Catherine C. Crone, MD[a,b,c,]*, Michael J. Marcangelo, MD[d],
John L. Shuster Jr, MD[e,f]

KEYWORDS

- Transplantation • Palliative care • Ventricular assist devices
- Psychiatric issues • Quality of life

Before 1972, patients with end-stage organ failure faced the prospect of inevitable physical decline and death. Extended survival became a possibility, however, when Medicare approved coverage for dialysis. Options were subsequently expanded by the growth of organ transplantation, which offered improvements in quality of life (QOL) and in survival rates. The demand for organ transplantation has grown to the point where 27,000 transplants were performed in the United States in 2008 and more than 100,000 patients are currently on transplant waiting lists.[1,2]

Despite the success of transplantation, its potential benefits are limited. Some patients are too ill to be listed for transplant, others are removed from the waiting list when they become too ill to survive transplant surgery, and still others do not

Dr Shuster has received research grant support from Abbott Laboratories, Eli Lilly and Co, and Johnson & Johnson.

[a] Department of Psychiatry, George Washington University, Washington, DC, USA
[b] Department of Psychiatry, Northern Virginia Branch, Virginia Commonwealth University, Richmond, VA, USA
[c] Department of Psychiatry, Inova Fairfax Hospital, 3300 Gallows Road, Falls Church, VA 22042, USA
[d] Department of Psychiatry and Behavioral Neuroscience, University of Chicago Hospitals, 5841 South Maryland Avenue, MC 3077, Chicago, IL 606037, USA
[e] Psychiatry and Medicine Program, Vanderbilt University School of Medicine, Nashville, TN, USA
[f] Department of Psychiatry, Vanderbilt University School of Medicine, 1601 23rd Avenue South, Nashville, TN 37232, USA
* Corresponding author. Department of Psychiatry, Inova Fairfax Hospital, 3300 Gallows Road, Falls Church, VA 22042.
E-mail address: cathy.crone@inova.org

Med Clin N Am 94 (2010) 1241–1254
doi:10.1016/j.mcna.2010.08.005
0025-7125/10/$ – see front matter © 2010 Elsevier Inc. All rights reserved.

medical.theclinics.com

survive the wait for a donor organ. For those who receive an organ, not all survive transplant surgery or the postoperative recovery period. For others, complications may limit long-term survival. Physicians who care for transplant patients need to be able to address end-of-life issues.

Given the realities of transplantation, both psychological concerns and psychiatric complications are to be expected. This article seeks to provide physicians with a review of psychiatric issues pertinent to the care of adults undergoing solid organ transplantation. Included is discussion of end-of-life issues and ventricular assist devices, the latter a growing option for patients with advanced heart failure.

PRETRANSPLANT EVALUATION

Patients undergo an extensive evaluation before being placed on a transplant list. This assessment consists of a comprehensive medical evaluation to determine a patient's need for transplantation, ability to survive transplant surgery, and likelihood of a successful outcome. A psychosocial evaluation is also performed by transplant social workers and mental health professionals, covering a broad range of topics (**Box 1**). Although they are used to assess transplant candidacy, psychosocial evaluations also serve other purposes (**Box 2**), most important is the ability to help develop an individualized treatment plan. Given the importance of adequate support before and after transplantation, family members and significant others are included in the psychosocial evaluation. Additional information from other mental health care providers, treatment facilities, and treating physicians may be gathered during the psychosocial evaluation when there are specific concerns about a patient's mental health, substance use history, and/or treatment adherence.

Although most patients approach transplantation with a mixture of hope and desperation, it is important to provide them with a realistic picture of this intervention.

Box 1
Content of the pretransplant psychosocial evaluation

1. History of end-stage organ disease (eg, onset, course, symptomatology)

2. Circumstances leading to transplant referral (eg, expected, emergent)

3. Attitude toward transplantation and level of interest

4. Expectations and concerns regarding transplantation

5. Understanding of transplant process (eg, risks, benefits, long-term prognosis)

6. History of treatment adherence (eg, with medications, appointments, diet)

7. History of other medical problems—and patient's experience with illness

8. Current/past psychiatric history, including cognitive difficulties

9. Current/past history of substance use/abuse

11. Family history of medical illnesses/psychiatric illnesses

12. Social history (eg, educational level, employment, living situation)

13. Support system (eg, family, friends, church members, others)

14. Mental status examination

Adapted from DiMartini A, Crone C, Fireman M, et al. Psychiatric aspects of organ transplantation in critical care. Crit Care Clin 2008;24:949–81; with permission.

Box 2
Psychosocial evaluation—goals/purpose

1. Foster the development of individualized treatment plans

2. Establish/strengthen patient-caregiver relationships

3. Encourage patient education and informed consent

4. Evaluate patient's coping skills and strengths/weaknesses

5. Assess treatment adherence and barriers to adherence

6. Diagnose psychiatric disorders/give treatment options

7. Identify the presence and availability of support systems

8. Provide patient with informational/support resources

9. Assist patients and families in the development of care plans

10. Participate in team selection of transplant candidates

Adapted from DiMartini A, Crone C, Fireman M, et al. Psychiatric aspects of organ transplantation in critical care. Crit Care Clin 2008;24:949–81; with permission.

Pretransplant evaluations allow teams to provide balanced information about the risks and benefits, to clarify potential misperceptions, and to address gaps in a patient's knowledge base. Given that patients may not qualify for a transplant, may not survive the waiting period, or may develop life-threatening complications, an initial discussion of end-of-life issues should be conducted. Addressing advance directives, treatment preferences, and palliative care early on in the process can minimize subsequent surprise and emotional trauma of patients and family members.

CONTROVERSIES REGARDING TRANSPLANT CANDIDACY
Substance Abuse

Substance abuse among patients considered for organ transplantation has long been a source of concern for both health care professionals and for those in the general population. This has been particularly true with liver transplantation, given the frequency with which alcohol and drug abuse contributes to end-stage liver disease. Experience has shown that many of these patients thrive after transplantation; therefore, the focus is on careful assessment of patients.[3,4] Candidacy for transplantation should be considered on a case-by-case basis and pretransplant evaluations should be performed by mental health specialists familiar with substance abuse and its aftermath. Complete assessment includes a thorough substance use history (including a discussion of continued use despite medical advice/serious health consequences, acceptance of a substance abuse diagnosis, feelings about long-term abstinence, and receptiveness to addictions treatment). Family or other supports should be included in the evaluation because they can play a critical role in the development and maintenance of abstinence or sobriety.

Studies have sought to identify risk factors for relapse after transplantation; most often the focus has been on patients with alcoholic liver disease. Although conclusions are limited by differences in study designs, assessment approaches, and patient populations, several factors (eg, prior experiences with rehabilitation programs, short-term abstinence before transplantation, presence of comorbid psychiatric disorders, family history of substance abuse) are predictive of greater relapse risk.[5–10] The presence of these risk factors, however, should not automatically rule out a patient from receiving a transplant. Rather, patients who are able to acknowledge their history of substance abuse and who are willing to work with the transplant team toward developing long-term abstinence should be considered. Use of random toxicology screens, implementation of behavioral contingency contracts, attendance at 12-step meetings, and enrollment in formal rehabilitation programs emphasize the importance of abstinence and/or sobriety. After transplantation, attention to possible relapse requires ongoing screening (through direct, nonjudgmental questioning about substance use).[11]

Treatment Adherence

To a great extent, successful transplantation is dependent on a patient's ability to adhere closely to a complex regimen (that includes daily medications, self-monitoring, lifestyle changes, clinical testing, and follow-up). Although transplant teams expect patients to make a lifelong commitment to treatment adherence, patients and their behavior often fall short of this goal. Unfortunately, nonadherence is a significant cause of acute and chronic rejection, graft loss, and death.[12] The challenge of treatment adherence is reflected in numerous publications, including a careful meta-analysis of more than 150 studies that found the average rate of immunosuppressant nonadherence was nearly one-fourth of patients each year.[13] Similar findings have been noted among studies and reviews of self-reported medication nonadherence.[12,14–16] Significant difficulties adhering to other behaviors (such as diet, exercise, monitoring of vital signs) have also been reported.[13]

Transplant teams are eager to predict which patients are at risk for nonadherence; however, attempts to identify risk factors are hampered by differences in study designs and the duration of follow-up.[13,17] Despite this, most studies suggest that a history of nonadherence, younger age, a longer period since transplant, and reduced social support are risk factors for treatment nonadherence.[12,13,15] The presence of reduced conscientiousness, low self-efficacy, poorer perceived health, and depression also seem to be potential risk factors.[13,15,18,19] Results regarding the impact of other factors (such as race, gender, education, socioeconomic status) have yielded mixed results. Addressing nonadherence among transplant patients requires an awareness that it is common for those confronting chronic medical conditions. Multidisciplinary approaches (that address educational, behavioral, psychological, and social support issues) are most efficacious. Open discussions with patients about potential concerns over medication side effects, financial issues, lifestyle changes, and other challenges should be encouraged even long after transplantation.

Psychiatric Disorders

Similar to patients with other forms of serious medical illness, patients referred for transplantation often have comorbid psychiatric disorders. Most often, these are anxiety or depressive disorders that predate the development of end-stage organ disease or arise secondary to stresses related to deteriorating health. Other forms of psychopathology (eg, bipolar disorder, personality disorders, or psychotic disorders) may be present. Active psychiatric disorders have the potential to interfere with a patient's ability to provide informed consent, to cooperate with caregivers, and to adhere to treatment, but no psychiatric disorder is an absolute contraindication to transplantation.

The course of the psychiatric disorder, the severity of symptoms, precipitating factors, and attitude toward and response to mental health treatment should each be evaluated. Collateral information from family members, mental health care providers, or treatment facilities assists with the assessment. Active thoughts of suicide or homicide, frequent acts of self-harm/mutilation, command hallucinations, paranoid delusions, or troubled relationships with caregivers should raise serious concerns about transplant candidacy. Such afflicted patients may require psychiatric care before being listed and should receive closer-than-usual follow-up after transplantation.

PRE-TRANSPLANT AND POST-TRANSPLANT PATIENT CARE
Pre-transplant Management of Anxiety and Depression

During the pretransplant period, the appearance of anxiety and depressive disorders is common.[20] Recognition of these disorders may be confounded by symptoms (eg, shortness of breath, fatigue, anorexia, insomnia) that result from end-stage organ failure. Questions regarding the presence of anhedonia, hopelessness, helplessness, guilt, or overwhelming fear that interferes with daily function can aid in diagnosis. Patients with depression may readily acknowledge irritability over sadness or tearfulness. Although anxiety and depression are understandable given patient stressors, it is important not to eschew the need for treatment with medications and psychotherapy.

Although an extensive discussion of transplant psychopharmacology is beyond the scope of this article, general recommendations regarding the use of antidepressants and anxiolytics in end-stage organ disease are readily available. Pharmacokinetic alterations call for the initiation of medications at lower-than-usual doses, with a gradual upwards titration until efficacy is achieved.[21] As a class, selective serotonin reuptake inhibitors are generally the best initial choice for an antidepressant (due to their tolerability, effectiveness, and minimal drug-drug interactions).[21] Serotonin norepinephrine reuptake inhibitors may induce hypertension; duloxetine, specifically, is not advised for patients with cirrhosis.[21] Mirtazapine may be helpful in patients with anorexia and insomnia; although bupropion can assist with smoking cessation, it can elevate blood pressure.[21] Because most antidepressants take several weeks to work, patients should be encouraged to take them daily and not simply as needed. Psychostimulants (given their rapid onset of action, overall tolerability, and safety even in the midst of serious medical illness) are another option for depressed patients.[21] Because methylphenidate and dextroamphetamine are short-acting agents, patients should be dosed twice a day, during the morning and then at noontime. They should not be used in patients with a history of substance abuse.

Benzodiazepines are a reasonable option for the treatment of anxiety in many patients, but caution is warranted in those with advanced lung disease, particularly in the presence of carbon dioxide retention. Judicious use can help to reduce dyspnea caused by anxiety.[22] Benzodiazepines should also be avoided in patients with hepatic encephalopathy, because such use can worsen their mental state. Lorazepam, oxazepam, and temazepam (which require only conjugation and not oxidative metabolism) are safer in patients with cirrhosis without encephalopathy. Buspirone, a nonbenzodiazepine alternative for the treatment of anxiety, should be prescribed daily at adequate doses over several weeks, because onset of action is delayed. Antidepressants also provide effective anxiolytic action.

Post-transplant Psychiatric Complications

Psychiatric disorders are common after transplantation and may represent a recurrence of a pretransplant diagnosis or arise de novo. Delirium often arises in the period soon after surgery as a result of infection, rejection, or side effects of immunosuppressants. Treatment of delirium is similar to that of delirium in nontransplant patients; treatment should focus on correction of the underlying cause. Although depression can develop at any time after transplantation, it may be somewhat more common in the first year after transplant. Independent of the organ transplanted, rates of depression approach 25%; depression may be more common in thoracic transplant recipients.[23] Anxiety is also prevalent after transplant (averaging 25%).[23] Posttraumatic stress disorder (a complex anxiety disorder characterized by intrusive thoughts, numbing, and hyperarousal) occurs in approximately 10% of transplant recipients.[24] Some of the factors evaluated before transplantation (eg, poor social support, history of a psychiatric disorder) seem to increase the risk of developing posttraumatic stress disorder.[24] Once the transplant team identifies a psychiatric disorder, prompt referral to a mental health professional affiliated with the team should follow. Selective serotonin reuptake inhibitors are better tolerated than are others classes of antidepressants and can be safely used in post-transplant patients. Sertraline, citalopram, and escitalopram, which have the fewest drug-drug interactions, are likely the safest choices.[25]

Neurotoxicity of Immunosuppressants

Immunosuppressants carry a significant risk of side effects, particularly in the early stages after transplantation when dosages are often at their highest. Although attention is often directed at the effects of glucocorticoids, cyclosporine and tacrolimus cause neurotoxicity in up to 60% of transplant recipients.[26] The calcineurin inhibitors can produce a wide range of signs and symptoms (including tremulousness, anxiety, delirium, and coma). Both can cause posterior reversible encephalopathy syndrome, a serious complication that can be manifest as a mental status change or a focal neurologic symptom.[21] Neurotoxicity from tacrolimus and cyclosporine can develop even at low or therapeutic drug levels. Reducing the drug dose, correction of metabolic disturbances (eg, an abnormal magnesium level), or switching from tacrolimus to cyclosporine may be needed if symptoms of neurotoxicity are significant.[21] Sirolimus seems to be associated with less neurotoxicity and may be a good alternative immunosuppressant for some patients.[27]

Quality of Life

The primary purpose of any medical procedure can either be to prolong life or to improve QOL. For patients with end-stage organ disease, transplantation extends life for the majority. The impact transplantation has on QOL is more complex because it varies with the organ involved and with each patient; part of the pretransplant selection process is aimed at identification of those patients who are likely to achieve improved physical and mental QOL after their transplant. Patients who undergo a liver transplant see improved QOL at 6 months; at 12 months, they often begin to see their mental health QOL ratings decline despite their improvement in overall health.[28] The decline continues until at least 5 years post-transplant.[29] Returning to work may contribute to improved QOL, although it may be that only patients with a good QOL are able to return to work. Regardless of which way the association goes, patients who return to work rate the quality of their mental health as higher than those who do not.[29]

Lung transplantation remains the most medically risky transplant procedure among organ transplantations. According to the United Network for Organ Sharing, the 5-year survival after lung transplantation is 47.3%.[1] Although this is an improvement over what their life expectancy would have been had they not undergone a transplant, the guarded prognosis implies that improved QOL must be part of the decision to perform lung transplantation. Patients who undergo lung transplantation see an improvement in their QOL, but this improvement takes longer to show itself than it does in heart transplant patients and it is not fully evident until 1 year after transplant.[30] One of the implications of this finding is that lung transplant patients may have high rates of psychiatric disorders shortly after transplant and, therefore, need significant psychiatric support during the first year of their recovery.

Patients who undergo transplant face long-term concerns as well. Chronic low-grade rejection can gradually erode graft function and eventually cause significant medical complications. Lung transplant recipients probably face the most serious and predictable of these complications, bronchiolitis obliterans. By 5 years post-transplant, approximately 40% of patients develop this complication,[31] and its presence is a significant factor in determining both physical and mental QOL.[32]

Similar problems can arise in other organs. For patients who have received a liver, recurrent hepatitis C remains a major problem. Patients who develop recurrent hepatitis C have a lower QOL and a higher rate of depression than do those who do not.[33] Because 95% of transplant recipients experience viral reactivation and as many as half go on to have a symptomatic recurrence, the risk for psychosocial problems after transplant for patients with hepatitis C is higher than in other groups. Likewise, heart transplant patients face cardiac allograph vasculopathy at rates that steadily increase and reach 43% 8 years after transplant.[34] Chronic rejection related to vasculopathy is one of many problems that contribute to a lower physical QOL 5 to 10 years after transplantation.[35]

RETRANSPLANTATION

Patients who face allograph failure may be candidates for retransplantation; however, survival is reduced for heart and liver recipients.[36,37] Given the shortage of available organs and the long waiting list that candidates face, patients do not automatically become candidates for retransplantation after repeat organ failure. In particular, if patients have suffered graft loss due to nonadherence, they should not be offered retransplantation unless there are well-understood extenuating circumstances. As an alternative, patients may be offered palliative care for their end-stage disease.

VENTRICULAR ASSIST DEVICES

When patients are not candidates for transplantation, alternatives are offered when possible. In recent years, left ventricular assist devices (LVADs) have become an increasingly available option to patients with advanced heart failure. Currently used as both a bridge to transplantation or as destination therapy, questions remain about the role these devices play in the continuum of care because of their high rates of complications and the often-limited lifespan associated with their use.

Guidelines for evaluation of LVAD candidates are generally similar to those for transplantation candidates.[38] The capacity to consent, a demonstrated ability to adhere to complex treatment regimens and to abstain from substance misuse, and the absence of active psychiatric disorders are all key components of the evaluation. One of the complexities encountered with many LVAD patients is the uncertainty as to whether or not the procedure is meant to be bridge-to-transplant or a destination therapy. Because destination therapy has been shown to decrease QOL but to extend lifespan,[39] this information needs to be conveyed to patients to facilitate their decision-making process. It has been argued that destination therapy is best seen as an end-of-life treatment, on the same spectrum as palliative care, and that advance care planning should occur at the same time that patients decide about their options related to LVAD placement.[40]

The cognitive assessment of patients who are candidates for LVAD placement is an essential part of the evaluation. Patients with chronic heart failure often have memory and attention deficits due to direct effects of their heart disease or its treatment. Because these deficits may have an impact on a patient's ability to provide informed consent, a cognitive evaluation should be performed on all LVAD candidates. A combination of Mini-Mental State Examination and an evaluation of frontal lobe functions (using tools, such as the frontal assessment battery,[41] which assesses factors, such as the ability to shift sets and to follow complex directions) helps provide a functional baseline.

Early experience suggests high rates of psychiatric disorders follow LVAD placement. Fully 83% of patients who received an LVAD required psychiatric consultation at one center.[42] Adjustment disorders, depressive disorders, and delirium were the most common diagnoses, and 16% of patients developed new-onset major depressive disorder after LVAD placement.[42] Many of the post-transplant psychiatric complications, including depression and anxiety, faced by transplant patients seem to be common post-LVAD placement.

Some of the psychosocial problems common among LVAD patients are different from those in the transplant population. The management of the device itself (eg, changing the battery and protecting the driveline as it enters the body) requires physical dexterity. Patients also need to have a charged battery available at all times; this can limit their mobility. The loss of control that such patients experience is one of the major barriers to a better QOL faced by LVAD recipients. For patients who have bridge-to-transplant devices, some of these chronic problems can be resolved with transplantation, but for destination patients and bridge patients who have long waits, these issues can compromise QOL. Overall, there is an improved QOL in patients who have survived for a year after LVAD placement.[43] Patients spend an average of 87% of their time outside of the hospital and their average New York Heart Association classification fell (in one study) from 4 to 2.[43] A caveat to these results is that only 29% of patients survived a year; however, if the device was meant as a destination device rather than as a bridge-to-transplant, the survival was 45%.[43]

PALLIATIVE CARE FOR TRANSPLANT PATIENTS

After the initial relief and elation that results from transplant listing, patients and families face the reality of an uncertain future awaiting a donor organ. Declining health, increasing disability, loss of independence, and the possibility of dying during the waiting period are significant challenges. Eventually, some individuals are removed from the waiting list. Given these realities, it is remarkable that formal relationships between transplant and palliative care teams are unusual.[44]

The clinician's task in working with transplant patients is to optimize their physical health and QOL, to maintain a sense of hope in the face of uncertainty, and to prepare them for the possibility that a donor organ will not arrive in time. Discussions initiated during the pretransplant evaluation regarding end-of-life issues should be periodically revisited. Families should be included in the discussions to help prepare them for potential loss. Assistance from pastoral care, social work, and mental health care specialists is often useful during this period.

It is always difficult to initiate discussions about end-of-life care, but perhaps it is never more so than when patients are candidates for transplantation. Patients and families balance the hope of prolonged survival, vastly improved health, and optimized

QOL against the possibility of decline and death. Because of the uncertainty produced by a scarcity of donor organs and the potential for pre- and post-transplant complications, many clinicians and patients decide not to invest the time or energy in these discussions. This is unfortunate, because patients eligible for organ transplantation typically value and desire symptom control, advance care planning, and information about the likely course of illness, although these needs often go unmet.[45,46]

Palliative care is care aimed at minimizing suffering and optimizing QOL when cure is no longer a reasonable expectation. The World Health Organization defines palliative care as "the active total care of patients whose disease is not responsive to curative treatment. Control of pain, of other symptoms, and of psychological, social, and spiritual problems, is paramount".[47] The word, *active*, underscores the fact that excellent palliative care involves the active pursuit of explicitly stated care goals, although these goals are different from those when acute illness strikes or when it is early in the course of chronic disease. Similarly, the word, *total*, indicates that palliative care takes a comprehensive, whole patient view of suffering and distress. In the United States, home-based hospice care (as defined by the Medicare hospice benefit) is the primary means of delivering palliative care to patients who qualify. The principles of palliative care, however, can be applied, as appropriate, independently of admission to a formal hospice program. The National Consensus Project for Quality Palliative Care's clinical practice guidelines state, "palliative care expands traditional disease-model medical treatments to include the goals of enhancing quality of life for patient and family, optimizing function, helping with decision making, and providing opportunities for personal growth. As such, it can be delivered concurrently with life-prolonging care or as the main focus of care."[48]

An understanding of the nature of palliative care can help clinicians dispel misconceptions that patients and families may have. Quality palliative care is not simply abandonment or benign neglect of patients with advanced and incurable illness. Although cure or disease eradication is no longer pursued and efforts to prolong life are intentionally considered in terms of their burden-to-benefit ratio, it is helpful to emphasize the active efforts and interventions that will be brought to bear on patient problems and distress. Symptoms and their relief are a focus of treatment. This often requires teaching patients to attend to symptoms and encouraging timely reporting, because symptoms may previously have been valued primarily for their diagnostic significance, if at all. It is often a great relief to patients to learn that symptom relief is a primary focus of palliative care. Psychosocial and spiritual concerns are also an area of emphasis, and the attention they receive can be of great value to patients and families. Explaining the value of palliative care and describing the treatment approach in terms that patients and families can understand are essential.

Palliative care programs focus care and intervention in several areas. First and foremost, patients and families are assured of nonabandonment. One of the things that patients facing the end of their lives fear most is that they will have to face the dying process alone. All too often, important others, including health care providers, withdraw from patients due to their discomfort witnessing the decline of someone they have cared for and cared about. It is important to face this discomfort and to prevent it from becoming a hindrance to presence, when patients need it most.

Symptom control (including treatment of pain, anxiety, depression, fatigue, nausea, constipation, and dyspnea) is a central task of palliative care. Patients are often reluctant to report symptoms, and multiple, interacting symptoms are the rule and not the exception in advanced disease. Systematic screening strategies (such as the Edmonton Symptom Assessment System) for multiple symptoms are helpful tools in this regard.[49]

Other palliative care interventions include assistance with life tasks (eg, attendance at important family events, giving gifts to family and friends, leaving a legacy, getting one's affairs in order). Repairing ruptured relationships, expressing gratitude and love, and saying goodbye to those closest to them are tasks that many patients undertake, although some may need help and advice to facilitate the process. Finally, palliative care providers assist with grief and bereavement, both anticipatory and reactive, in patients and families. Hospice programs generally offer bereavement aftercare for surviving family members. Excellent palliative care helps preserve hope and morale in the setting of incurable illness, preserves a sense of dignity, and can enable occasions for healing and wholeness, even when advancing illness cannot be reversed.

Eligibility for hospice care is determined by the Medicare hospice benefit, established in 1984. To be eligible for hospice care, patients must have an advanced and life-limiting disease, opt for palliative goals of care, and be certified as terminally ill. Terminal illness is defined as an illness with a life expectancy of 6 months or less, as judged by two physicians, assuming the illness runs its typical course. This leads to obvious barriers to care for patients who are listed for an organ transplant who might benefit from hospice care. End-of-life prognostication is difficult at best but becomes even more problematic in the setting of organ transplantation. A primary goal of transplantation is to add years to a patient's life, but most transplant-eligible patients would be hospice eligible without a new organ or a similarly aggressive intervention. Hospice programs are often reluctant to admit patients whose treatment is so complex and so explicitly aimed at life extension (perceived as philosophically in conflict with hospice philosophy). Additionally, the expense of pretransplant care is typically far in excess of the per diem reimbursement for hospice care. The requirement for patients to sign a hospice election form explicitly acknowledging terminal illness is itself a barrier. Although a patient's prognosis may make hospice care appropriate, a patient and family may perceive the explicit shift in care goals as tantamount to giving up hope.

The philosophic approach of palliative care can be implemented without referral to a formal hospice program. Specific attention to palliative goals of care (eg, symptom control, maintenance and repair of meaningful interpersonal relationships, spiritual and existential peace) can give great relief, with or without formal palliative care consultation.

Hospice eligibility concerns aside, one could ask, "When should a patient with advanced and potentially fatal illness be referred for palliative care? At the time of initial diagnosis? As clinical milestones of advanced disease are reached or passed? When all curative options are exhausted?" Patients who are deemed ineligible for transplant of a vital organ should be offered palliative care/hospice. Additionally, given that the majority of potentially eligible patients never receive a donor organ, it is reasonable to offer palliative care and even hospice care to patients who are awaiting transplant. Rossaro and colleagues[50] have described such an approach, which requires a high degree of collaboration between transplant and hospice care teams. Patients suffering from vital organ failure can continue to receive pretransplant care and monitoring while benefiting from the comprehensive palliative treatment approach offered by hospice. If a suitable graft becomes available, patients can revoke the hospice benefit and pursue transplantation. If a donor organ is never identified, patients and families benefit from palliative care as the trajectory of advancing illness moves toward death, avoiding the difficulties of referral in the last few days of life. This integrated approach is in sharp contrast to the either/or paradigm most commonly used for patients who are transplant candidates and should be practical in most transplantation centers. Although no published data are available to assess the impact of such an integrated approach on pretransplant survival, there is no reason to expect an adverse effect.

Perhaps the most challenging aspect of palliative care for transplant patients is how to initiate discussions about palliative and end-of-life care and negotiate goals of care. Published guidelines and advice for breaking bad news and facilitating these emotionally charged discussions are plentiful.[51,52] Palliative care specialists recognize that negotiating the goals of care is one of the core skills in excellent end-of-life care and is the key to successful implementation of a palliative care plan.[53]

An approach to negotiating goals of care should incorporate the steps outlined in **Box 3**. Setting explicit goals of care is valuable because goals guide care, whether or not they are explicitly stated or agreed on. Explicit goal-setting also shapes family expectations and helps families plan and set priorities.[53] In setting palliative care goals, patients' expressed wishes and preferences should take precedence, because target outcomes are typically more subjective. It is important to recognize that serial discussions about goals of care are usually necessary in the setting of a dynamic and advancing disease. Appropriate goals (including life extension, improvement or preservation of function, provision of comfort, optimization of QOL, and easing the dying process) should be considered. It is also important to find the right balance in facilitating these discussions, being thorough and realistic in the presentation of the clinical situation without being coercive or inappropriately paternalistic. One should be prepared for patients and families to choose treatment options that a clinician might not choose or even recommend. Unless patients are clearly being harmed by

---

Box 3
Eleven steps for negotiating goals of care

1. Reach a consensus among the treating team before the conference (eg, prognosis, which treatments are reasonable to offer, who will moderate the conference).

2. Determine agency (ie, who speaks for the patient—patient or proxy).

3. Set up a family conference. Make formal introductions; set an explicit agenda.

4. Determine patient's (or the proxy/surrogate's) understanding of the clinical situation.

5. Determine patient's wishes, preferences, and values relevant to the clinical situation. If a patient cannot speak for him/herself, is an advance directive available as a guide? If not, clarify for the proxy that he/she is speaking for the patient as the person who best knows how the patient's wishes, preferences, and values would guide decision-making.

6. Explain the reality of the clinical situation in clear, nontechnical terms, being tactful but clear. Provide the rationale for any recommendations against a treatment option and suggest reasonable alternatives.

7. Link decisions about goals with patient's wishes, preferences, and values. Relate decisions about goals to expressed wishes (or the proxy's best estimate). The overall goal is to honor a patient's wishes and preferences. Express goals in balanced terms (eg, what will be avoided or foregone, what will be pursued or provided).

8. Formulate a consensus plan for care and document this in the medical record.

9. Anticipate likely events or complications and outline contingency plans.

10. Create follow-up plans: When will decisions be implemented? How will the response to treatment be agreed on be monitored?

11. Follow through—say what you will do. Do what you say. Follow-up as promised.

the decision or a requested treatment is blatantly unrealistic or contraindicated, clinicians should err on the side of respecting patients' wishes, preferences, and values.

REFERENCES

1. Wolfe RA, Roys EC, Merion RM. Trends in organ donation and transplantation in the United States, 1999–2008. Am J Transplant 2010;10:961–72.
2. United network for organ sharing. Available at: http://www.unos.org. Accessed May 31, 2010.
3. Burra P, Senzolo M, Adam R, et al. Liver transplantation for alcoholic liver disease in Europe: a study from the ELTR (European Liver Transplant Registry). Am J Transplant 2010;10:138–48.
4. Lucey MR. Liver transplantation for alcoholic liver disease. Clin Liver Dis 2007;11: 283–9.
5. Tandon P, Goodman KJ, Wong WW, et al. A shorter duration of pre-transplant abstinence predicts problem drinking after liver transplantation. Am J Gastroenterol 2009;104:1700–6.
6. Dew MA, DiMartini AF, Steel J, et al. Meta-analysis of risk for relapse to substance use after transplantation of the liver or other solid organs. Liver Transpl 2008;14: 159–72.
7. Kotlyar DS, Burke A, Campbell MS, et al. A critical review of candidacy for orthotopic liver transplantation in alcoholic liver disease. Am J Gastroenterol 2008;103: 734–43.
8. De Gottardi A, Spahr L, Gelez P, et al. A simple score for predicting alcohol relapse after liver transplantation: results from 387 patients over 15 years. Arch Intern Med 2007;167:1183–8.
9. Kelly M, Chick J, Gribble R, et al. Predictors of relapse to harmful alcohol after orthotopic liver transplantation. Alcohol Alcohol 2006;41:278–83.
10. Miguet M, Monnet E, Vanlemmens C, et al. Predictive factors of alcohol relapse after orthotopic liver transplantation for alcoholic liver disease. Gastroenterol Clin Biol 2004;28:845–51.
11. DiMartini A, Day N, Dew MA, et al. Alcohol use following liver transplantation: a comparison of follow-up methods. Psychosomatics 2001;42:55–62.
12. Morissey PE, Flynn ML, Lin S. Medication noncompliance and its implications in transplant recipients. Drugs 2007;67:1463–81.
13. Dew MA, DiMartini AF, De Vito Dabbs A, et al. Rates and risk factors for nonadherence to the medical regimen after adult solid organ transplantation. Transplantation 2007;15:858–73.
14. Gordon EJ, Prohaska TR, Gallant MP, et al. Adherence to immunosuppression: a prospective diary study. Transplant Proc 2007;39:3081–5.
15. Denhaerynck K, Dobbels F, Cleemput I, et al. Prevalence, consequences, and determinants of nonadherence in adult renal transplant patients: a literature review. Transpl Int 2005;18:1121–33.
16. Butler JA, Roderick P, Mullee M, et al. Frequency and impact of nonadherence to immunosuppressants after renal transplantation: a systematic review. Transplantation 2004;77:769–89.
17. Dew MA, DiMartini AF. The incidence of nonadherence after organ transplant: ensuring that our efforts at counting really count. Liver Transpl 2006;12:1736–40.
18. Dobbels F, Vanhaecke J, Dupont L, et al. Pretransplant predictors of posttransplant adherence and clinical outcome: an evidence base for pretransplant psychosocial screening. Transplantation 2009;87:1497–504.

19. Jindal RM, Neff RT, Abbott KC, et al. Association between depression and non-adherence in recipients of kidney transplants: analysis of the United States renal data system. Transplant Proc 2009;41:3662–6.
20. DiMartini A, Crone C, Fireman M, et al. Psychiatric aspects of organ transplantation in critical care. Crit Care Clin 2008;24:949–81.
21. DiMartini AF, Crone CC, Fireman M. Organ transplantation. In: Ferrando SJ, Levenson JL, Owen JA, editors. Clinical manual of psychopharmacology in the medically Ill. Arlington (VA): American Psychiatric Publishing; 2010. p. 469–99.
22. Thompson WL, Smolin YL. Respiratory disorders. In: Ferrando SJ, Levenson JL, Owen JA, editors. Clinical manual of psychopharmacology in the medically Ill. Arlington (VA): American Psychiatric Publishing; 2010. p. 213–35.
23. Dew MA, Kormos RL, DiMartini AF, et al. Prevalence and risk of depression and anxiety-related disorders during the first three years after heart transplantation. Psychosomatics 2001;42:300–13.
24. Stukas AA Jr, Dew MA, Switzer GE, et al. PTSD in heart transplant recipients and their primary family caregivers. Psychosomatics 1999;40:212–21.
25. Crone CC, Gabriel GM. Treatment of anxiety and depression in transplant patients: pharmacokinetic considerations. Clin Pharmacokinet 2004;43:361–94.
26. Bechstein WO. Neurotoxicity of calcineurin inhibitors: impact and clinical management. Transpl Int 2000;13:313–26.
27. Heinrich TW, Marcangelo M. Psychiatric issues in solid organ transplantation. Harv Rev Psychiatry 2009;17:398–406.
28. Tome S, Wells JT, Said A, et al. Quality of life after liver transplantation. A systematic review. J Hepatol 2008;48:567–77.
29. Bownik H, Saab S. Health-related quality of life after liver transplantation for adult recipients. Liver Transpl 2009;15(Suppl 2):S42–9.
30. Myaskovsky L, Dew MA, McNulty ML, et al. Trajectories of change in quality of life in 12-month survivors of lung or heart transplant. Am J Transplant 2006;6: 1939–47.
31. Kunsebeck HW, Kugler C, Fischer S, et al. Quality of life and bronchiolitis obliterans syndrome in patients after lung transplantation. Prog Transplant 2007;17(2): 136–41.
32. Vermuelen KM, can de Bij W, Erasmus ME, et al. Long-term health-related quality of life after lung transplantation: different predictors for different dimensions. J Heart Lung Transplant 2007;26(2):188–93.
33. Singh N, Gayowksi T, Wagener MM, et al. Quality of life, functional status, and depression in male liver transplant recipients with recurrent viral hepatitis C. Transplantation 1999;67(1):69–72.
34. Taylor DO, Edwards LB, Boucek MM, et al. Registry of the international society for heart and lung transplantation: twenty-third official adult heart transplantation report—2006. J Heart Lung Transplant 2006;25(8):869–79.
35. Grady KL, Naftel DC, Young JB, et al. Patterns and predictors of physical functional disability at 5 to 10 years after heart transplantation. J Heart Lung Transplant 2007;26(11):1182–91.
36. Tjang YS, Tenderich G, Hornik L, et al. Cardiac retransplantation in adults: an evidence-based systematic review. Thorac Cardiovasc Surg 2008;56(6):323–7.
37. Biggins SW, Beldecos A, Rabkin JM. Retransplantation for hepatic allograft failure: prognostic modeling and ethical considerations. Liver Transpl 2002; 8(4):313–22.
38. Marcus P. Left ventricular assist devices: psychosocial challenges in the elderly. Ann Thorac Surg 2009;88(5):e48–9.

39. Wray J, Hallas CN, Banner NR. Quality of life and psychological well-being during and after left ventricular assist device support. Clin Transplant 2007;21(5):622–7.

40. Dudzinski DM. Ethics guidelines for destination therapy. Ann Thorac Surg 2006; 81(4):1185–8.

41. Dubois B, Slachevsky A, Litvan I, et al. The FAB: a frontal assessment battery at bedside. Neurology 2000;55(11):1621–6.

42. Shapiro PA, Levin HR, Oz MC. Left ventricular assist devices. Psychosocial burden and implications for heart transplant programs. Gen Hosp Psychiatry 1996;19(Suppl 6). 30S–35S.

43. Allen JG, Weiss ES, Schaffer JM. Quality of life and functional status in patients surviving 12 months after left ventricular assist device implantation. J Heart Lung Transplant 2010;29(3):278–85.

44. Molmenti EP, Dunn GP. Transplantation and palliative care: the convergence of two seemingly opposite realities. Surg Clin North Am 2005;85:373–82.

45. Davison SN. End-of-life care preference and needs: perceptions of patients with chronic kidney disease. Clin J Am Soc Nephrol 2010;5:195–204.

46. Steinhauser KE, Christakis NA, Clipp EC, et al. Factors considered important at the end of life by patients, family, physicians, and other care providers. JAMA 2000;284:2476–82.

47. World Health Organization. Cancer pain relief and palliative care: report of a WHO expert committee. World Health Organ Tech Rep Ser 1990;804:1–75.

48. National consensus project for quality palliative care: clinical practice guidelines for quality palliative care, 2nd edition. National Consensus Project for Quality Palliative Care, 2009. Available at: http://www.nationalconsensusproject.org/guideline.pdf. Accessed June 10, 2010.

49. Bruera E, Kuehn N, Miller MJ, et al. The edmonton symptom assessment system (ESAS): a simple method for the assessment of palliative care patients. J Palliat Care 1991;7:6–9.

50. Rossaro L, Troppmann C, McVicar JP, et al. A strategy for the simultaneous provision of pre-operative palliative care for patients awaiting liver transplantation. Transpl Int 2004;17:473–5.

51. Baile WF, Buckman R, Lenzi R, et al. SPIKES—A six-step protocol for delivering bad news: application to the patient with cancer. Oncologist 2000;5:302–11.

52. Buckman R. Breaking bad news: why is it still so difficult? BMJ 1984;288:1597–9.

53. EPEC project (the project to educate physicians on end-of-life care): EPEC participant's handbook: module 7, goals of care. The Robert Wood Johnson Foundation, 1999. Available at: http://endoflife.northwestern.edu/goals_of_care/module7.pdf. Accessed June 10, 2010.

Index

Note: Page numbers of article titles are in **boldface** type.

A

Abuse, reporting of, 1229–1230
Acamprosate, for alcohol dependence, 1180
Acetylcholinesterase inhibitors, for dementia, 1111–1112
S-Adenosylmethionine (SAMe), 1155–1157
Adherence, to treatment, 1081–1082, 1206–1209, 1242
Advanced directives, 1233–1234
Agitation, in dementia, 1112
Agnosia, in Alzheimer disease, 1109
Alcohol use disorder, 1170–1180
    acute intoxication in, 1171–1172
    acute stages of, 1170
    dependence in, 1180
    epidemiology of, 1170
    late stages of, 1170–1171
    mechanism of action of, 1170–1171
    tolerance in, 1170–1171
Alcohol-Withdrawal Syndrome Scale, 1174
Alpha$_2$-adrenergic receptor agonists, for alcohol withdrawal, 1177–1180
Alprazolam, 1148
    for anxiety disorders, 1133–1134
    intoxication with, 1184, 1187
    pharmacology of, 1186
Alzheimer disease, 1108–1109, 1111–1112
Amnesia, in Alzheimer disease, 1109
Amphetamines, abuse of, 1189
Anorexia, 1219
Anticholinergics
    abuse of, 1198
    delirium due to, 1107
    for forgetfulness, 1220
Anticonvulsants
    for alcohol withdrawal, 1176–1177
    for mood disorders, 1150–1152
Antidepressants, 1144–1147
    atypical, 1145–1146
    augmenting agents with, 1147
    for anxiety disorders, 1132–1133
    for dementia, 1112
    for insomnia, 1218

Med Clin N Am 94 (2010) 1255–1270
doi:10.1016/S0025-7125(10)00181-1
0025-7125/10/$ – see front matter © 2010 Elsevier Inc. All rights reserved.

United States Postal Service
Statement of Ownership, Management, and Circulation
(All Periodicals Publications Except Requester Publications)

1. Publication Title	2. Publication Number	3. Filing Date
Medical Clinics of North America	3 3 7 - 3 4 0	9/15/10

4. Issue Frequency	5. Number of Issues Published Annually	6. Annual Subscription Price
Jan, Mar, May, Jul, Sep, Nov	6	$204.00

7. Complete Mailing Address of Known Office of Publication (Not printer) (Street, city, county, state, and ZIP+4®)

Elsevier Inc.
360 Park Avenue South
New York, NY 10010-1710

Contact Person
Stephen Bushing
Telephone (Include area code)
215-239-3688

8. Complete Mailing Address of Headquarters or General Business Office of Publisher (Not printer)

Elsevier Inc., 360 Park Avenue South, New York, NY 10010-1710

9. Full Names and Complete Mailing Addresses of Publisher, Editor, and Managing Editor (Do not leave blank)

Publisher (Name and complete mailing address)

Kim Murphy, Elsevier, Inc., 1600 John F. Kennedy Blvd. Suite 1800, Philadelphia, PA 19103-2899

Editor (Name and complete mailing address)

Rachel Glover, Elsevier, Inc., 1600 John F. Kennedy Blvd. Suite 1800, Philadelphia, PA 19103-2899

Managing Editor (Name and complete mailing address)

Catherine Bewick, Elsevier, Inc., 1600 John F. Kennedy Blvd. Suite 1800, Philadelphia, PA 19103-2899

10. Owner (Do not leave blank. If the publication is owned by a corporation, give the name and address of the corporation immediately followed by the names and addresses of all stockholders owning or holding 1 percent or more of the total amount of stock. If not owned by a corporation, give the names and addresses of the individual owners. If owned by a partnership or other unincorporated firm, give its name and address as well as those of each individual owner. If the publication is published by a nonprofit organization, give its name and address.)

Full Name	Complete Mailing Address
Wholly owned subsidiary of	4520 East-West Highway
Reed/Elsevier, US holdings	Bethesda, MD 20814

11. Known Bondholders, Mortgagees, and Other Security Holders Owning or Holding 1 Percent or More of Total Amount of Bonds, Mortgages, or Other Securities. If none, check box ☐ None

Full Name	Complete Mailing Address
N/A	

12. Tax Status (For completion by nonprofit organizations authorized to mail at nonprofit rates) (Check one)
The purpose, function, and nonprofit status of this organization and the exempt status for federal income tax purposes:
☐ Has Not Changed During Preceding 12 Months
☐ Has Changed During Preceding 12 Months (Publisher must submit explanation of change with this statement)

PS Form 3526, September 2007 (Page 1 of 3 (Instructions Page 3)) PSN 7530-01-000-9931 PRIVACY NOTICE: See our Privacy policy in www.usps.com

13. Publication Title	14. Issue Date for Circulation Data Below
Medical Clinics of North America	September 2010

15. Extent and Nature of Circulation		Average No. Copies Each Issue During Preceding 12 Months	No. Copies of Single Issue Published Nearest to Filing Date
a. Total Number of Copies (Net press run)		3552	3312
b. Paid Circulation (By Mail and Outside the Mail)	(1) Mailed Outside-County Paid Subscriptions Stated on PS Form 3541. (Include paid distribution above nominal rate, advertiser's proof copies, and exchange copies)	1574	1457
	(2) Mailed In-County Paid Subscriptions Stated on PS Form 3541 (Include paid distribution above nominal rate, advertiser's proof copies, and exchange copies)		
	(3) Paid Distribution Outside the Mails Including Sales Through Dealers and Carriers, Street Vendors, Counter Sales, and Other Paid Distribution Outside USPS®	845	925
	(4) Paid Distribution by Other Classes Mailed Through the USPS (e.g. First-Class Mail®)		
c. Total Paid Distribution (Sum of 15b (1), (2), (3), and (4))	▶	2419	2382
d. Free or Nominal Rate Distribution (By Mail and Outside the Mail)	(1) Free or Nominal Rate Outside-County Copies Included on PS Form 3541	148	109
	(2) Free or Nominal Rate In-County Copies Included on PS Form 3541		
	(3) Free or Nominal Rate Copies Mailed at Other Classes Through the USPS (e.g. First-Class Mail)		
	(4) Free or Nominal Rate Distribution Outside the Mail (Carriers or other means)		
e. Total Free or Nominal Rate Distribution (Sum of 15d (1), (2), (3) and (4))	▶	148	109
f. Total Distribution (Sum of 15c and 15e)	▶	2567	2491
g. Copies not Distributed (See instructions to publishers #4 (page #3))	▶	985	821
h. Total (Sum of 15f and g)	▶	3552	3312
i. Percent Paid (15c divided by 15f times 100)		94.23%	95.62%

16. Publication of Statement of Ownership

If the publication is a general publication, publication of this statement is required. Will be printed ☐ Publication not required
in the November 2010 issue of this publication.

17. Signature and Title of Editor, Publisher, Business Manager, or Owner	Date
Stephen R. Bushing — Fulfillment/Inventory Specialist	September 15, 2010

Stephen R. Bushing – Fulfillment/Inventory Specialist

I certify that all information furnished on this form is true and complete. I understand that anyone who furnishes false or misleading information on this form or who omits material or information requested on the form may be subject to criminal sanctions (including fines and imprisonment) and/or civil sanctions (including civil penalties).

PS Form 3526, September 2007 (Page 2 of 3)

Moving?

Make sure your subscription moves with you!

To notify us of your new address, find your **Clinics Account Number** (located on your mailing label above your name), and contact customer service at:

Email: journalscustomerservice-usa@elsevier.com

800-654-2452 (subscribers in the U.S. & Canada)
314-447-8871 (subscribers outside of the U.S. & Canada)

Fax number: 314-447-8029

Elsevier Health Sciences Division
Subscription Customer Service
3251 Riverport Lane
Maryland Heights, MO 63043

*To ensure uninterrupted delivery of your subscription, please notify us at least 4 weeks in advance of move.

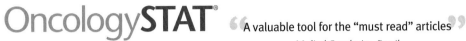

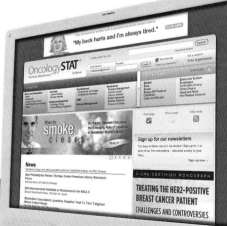